Viva In Anatomy

(Part One)

Fourth Edition

Viva In Anatomy

(Part One)

General Anatomy
Upper Limb
Lower Limb
and
Thorax

By
A. Yadav MS

JAYPEE BROTHERS
MEDICAL PUBLISHERS (P) LTD

New Delhi • Ahmedabad • Bengaluru • Chennai • Hyderabad • Kochi • Kolkata • Lucknow • Mumbai • Nagpur

Published by

Jitendar P Vij
Jaypee Brothers Medical Publishers (P) Ltd
EMCA House, 23/23B Ansari Road, Daryaganj, **New Delhi** 110 002, India
Phones: +91-11-23272143, 23272703, 23282021, 23245672
Fax: +91-11-23276490, +91-11-23245683
e-mail: jaypee@jaypeebrothers.com
Visit our website: www.jaypeebrothers.com

Branches

- 2/B, Akruti Society, Jodhpur Gam Road Satellite
  Ahmedabad 440 009 (MS) Phone: +91-79-30988717
- 202 Batavia Chambers, 8 Kumara Krupa Road
  Kumara Park East, **Bangalore** 560 001
  Phones: +91-80-22285971, +91-80-22382956, +91-80-30614073
  Tele Fax : +91-80-22281761 e-mail: jaypeebc@bgl.vsnl.net.in
- 282 IIIrd Floor, Khaleel Shirazi Estate, Fountain Plaza
  Pantheon Road, **Chennai** 600 008, Phones: +91-44-28262665, 28269897
  Fax: +91-44-28262331 e-mail: jpchen@eth.net
- 4-2-1067/1-3, 1st Floor, Balaji Building, Ramkote Cross Road
  Hyderabad 500 095, Phones: +91-40-55610020, +91-40-24758498
  Fax: +91-40-24758499 e-mail: jpmedpub@rediffmail.com
- 1A Indian Mirror Street, Wellington Square
  Kolkata 700 013, Phones: +91-33-22456075, +91-33-22451926
  Fax: +91-33-22456075 e-mail: jpbcal@cal.vsnl.net.in
- 106 Amit Industrial Estate, 61 Dr SS Rao Road Near MGM Hospital,
  Parel, **Mumbai** 400 012, Phones: +91-22-24124863, 24104532, 30926896
  Fax: +91-22-24160828 e-mail: jpmedpub@bom7.vsnl.net.in
- "KAMALPUSHPA" 38, Reshimbag Opp. Mohota Science College,
  Umred Road **Nagpur** 440 009 (MS)
  Phone: +91-712-3945220, e-mail: jpmednagpur@rediffmail.com

Viva in Anatomy

First Edition : 1984
Second Edition : 1987
Third Edition : 1990
Fourth Edition : 1999
Reprint : 2003
Reprint : 2006
Reprint **: 2008**

ISBN 81-7179-698-2

Typeset at JPBMP typesetting unit

Printed at Rajkamal Electric Press, Plot No. 2, Phase-IV, Kundli, Haryana.

Dedicated
to
My Teachers
and
Parents

Preface to the Fourth Edition

Appearance of another edition in a quick succession speaks itself of the great popularity and adaptation by the students. This edition has been thoroughly revised and a large number of clinically related questions added while retaining the original objective of the book i.e. to let the medical students have some basic concept of anatomy and equip themsevles better than others for the examinations.

The author sincerely hopes that this thoroughly revised edition which is quite handy and updated, will be of immense utility to the students. The author would feel duly rewarded if this book could be of some help in brushing up the knowledge of the students of anatomy.

Last but not the least, is the author's gratitude to the publishers Jaypee Brothers Medical Publishers for all the help rendered in publication of this book in record time.

Readers candid comments are most welcome.

A. Yadav

Preface to the First Edition

Several techniques may be applied to test the knowledge of examinees. However, Viva-voce continues to be the most popular technique. Whatever a student learns he or she is judged by his or her ability to reply questions in oral test.

This book is not intended to be a substitute for standard text books but aims to equip the students with probable questions and their exact answers, so that they perform better than who just grope in dark. The questions are selected from author's experience to enable students to know important and relevant aspects of each topic and perform well in viva-voce. The book has also incorporated the clinically related questions.

The author will be duly rewarded if the book comes upto the expectations of examinees and those who want to have some basic concept on anatomy.

I express my heart felt gratitude to all those friends and well wishers for their encouragement and guidance in the preparation of this book without which it would not have been possible to bring out the book.

My thanks are also to the publishers who spared no efforts to bring out this book as quickly as possible.

Comments and suggestions are welcome for improvement in subsequent editions through the publishers.

A. Yadav

Contents

General Anatomy

1. **Musculoskeletal System** ---------- *1*
   Osteology ---------- *1*
   Cartilage ---------- *5*
   Arthrology ---------- *6*
   Myology ---------- *9*
2. **Circulatory System** ---------- *12*
3. **Lymphatic System** ---------- *15*
4. **Nervous System** ---------- *17*

Upper Limb

1. **Bones of Upper Limb** ---------- *23*
   Clavicle ---------- *23*
   Scapula ---------- *24*
   Humerus ---------- *26*
   Radius and Ulna ---------- *28*
   Bones of Hand ---------- *30*
2. **Joints of Upper Limb** ---------- *32*
   Shoulder Joint ---------- *32*
   Shoulder Girdle ---------- *34*
   Elbow Joint ---------- *35*
   Cubital Fossa ---------- *36*
   Radio-ulnar Joint ---------- *38*
   Wrist Joint ---------- *39*
   Joints of Hand ---------- *40*
3. **Axilla** ---------- *43*
4. **Arteries of Upper Limb** ---------- *44*
   Venous Drainage of Upper Limb ---------- *48*
   Lymphatic Drainage of Upper Limb ---------- *49*
5. **Breast** ---------- *49*
6. **Brachial Plexus** ---------- *55*
   Radial Nerve ---------- *59*
   Musculocutaneous Nerve ---------- *61*
   Median Nerve ---------- *62*
   Ulnar Nerve ---------- *64*

7. **Scapular Spaces** ---------- 66
8. **Spaces of The Hand** ---------- 67

Lower Limb

1. **Bones of Lower Limb** ---------- 70
   Hip Bone ---------- 70
   Femur ---------- 73
   Tibia and Fibula ---------- 75
   Patella ---------- 77
   Bones of Foot ---------- 77
2. **Joints of Lower Limb** ---------- 79
   Hip Joint ---------- 79
   Knee Joint ---------- 82
   Ankle Joint ---------- 87
   Tibiofibular Joints ---------- 89
   Joints of Foot ---------- 89
   Arches of Foot ---------- 90
3. **Thigh** ---------- 93
   Femoral Triangle ---------- 95
   Adductor Canal ---------- 98
   Popliteal Fossa ---------- 98
4. **Gluteal Region** ---------- 99
5. **Leg and Foot** ---------- 101
6. **Arterial Supply of Lower Limb** ---------- 104
7. **Venous Drainage** ---------- 107
8. **Lymphatic Drainage of Lower Limb** ---------- 108
9. **Nerves of Lower Limb** ---------- 109
   Lumbar Plexus ---------- 109
   Sacral Plexus ---------- 111

Thorax

1. **Thoracic Cage** ---------- 118
   Ribs ---------- 119
   Sternum ---------- 123
   Thoracic Vertebrae ---------- 125
   Intercostal Spaces ---------- 125
2. **Pleurae** ---------- 130
3. **Lower Respiratory Tract** ---------- 133
   Trachea ---------- 133

Bronchi ---------- *137*

Lungs ---------- *137*

4. Mediastinum ---------- ***141***

5. Pericardium ---------- ***144***

6. Heart ---------- ***146***

Blood Supply of Heart ---------- *150*

Conducting System of the Heart ---------- *152*

7. Major Blood Vessels of Thorax ---------- ***154***

Superior Vena Cava ---------- ***154***

Pulmonary Trunk and Arteries ---------- *155*

Aorta ---------- *156*

Azygous and Hemiazygous Veins ---------- *158*

8. Oesophagus ---------- ***158***

9. Thoracic Duct ---------- ***161***

10. Sympathetic Trunk ---------- ***162***

11. Phrenic Nerves ---------- ***164***

General Anatomy

MUSCULOSKELETAL SYSTEM

OSTEOLOGY

Q. What are the subdivisions of skeleton?

Ans. The skeleton is divided into:

(a) *Axial skeleton:* It is central bony frame work, e.g., skull, vertebral column and thoracic cage.

(b) *Appendicular skeleton:* Formed by peripheral bones of the limbs.

Q. How the bones are classified according to shape?

Ans. (a) *Long bones:* Characterized by elongated tubular shaft, having a central medullary cavity and expanded articular ends (epiphyses), e.g., humerus, radius, femur etc.

(b) *Smaller long bones:* They have only one epiphyses, e.g., metacarpals, metatarsal.

(c) *Short bones:* They are cuboid, cuneiform, scaphoid or trapezoid in shape, e.g., carpal and tarsal bones.

(d) *Flat bones:* Like shallow plates, e.g., ribs, scapula and bones of cranial vault.

(e) *Irregular bones:* Includes those bones which cannot be assigned to any of above groups, e.g., hip bone, vertebrae etc.

(f) *Pneumatic bones:* They contain air spaces and are lined by mucous membrane, e.g., maxilla.

(g) *Accessory bones:* These are sometimes present in relation to limbs and skull bones.

Q. What are the functions of the bones?

Ans. (a) Provide shape and size to body

(b) Provide attachment to muscles, ligaments and tendons

(c) Protect vital organs

(d) Resist compression and tension stresses due to collagen tissue in bones
(e) Act as store house for calcium and phosphorus
(f) Act as a system of levers for movements by muscles
(g) Ear ossicles help in audition
(h) Bone marrow has blood forming function
(i) Reticuloendothelial cells of marrow are phagocytic and have a role in immune reactions
(j) Air sinuses in skull provide resonance to the voice.

Q. What are sites where red bone marrow is present in adults?

Ans. Proximal ends of femur and humerus, ribs, sternum, skull, vertebrae and hip bone.

Q. What is Anthropometry?

Ans. It is the study of variation in dimensions and bodily proportions of various bones in different races and with age and sex in a single race.

Q. What are the parts of long bone?

Ans. (a) *Epiphysis:* Ends of a long bone which ossifies from secondary centres.
(b) *Diaphysis:* Shaft of a long bone which ossifies from a primary centre. It consists of an outer cortex of compact bone and inner medullary cavity filled with bone marrow.
(c) *Metaphysis:* The epiphysial ends of diaphysis. It is the zone of active growth of bone.
(d) *Epiphysial plate of cartilage:* It separates metaphysis and epiphysis. Proliferation of this cartilaginous plate leads to lengthwise growth of bone.

Q. What are the different types of epiphyses?

Ans. (a) *Pressure epiphysis:* Articular and takes part in transmission of weight, e.g., head of femur, lower end of radius, medial end of clavicle.
(b) *Traction epiphysis:* Non articular. One or more tendon is attached to it which exerts a traction on it, e.g., trochanters of femur.
(c) *Atavistic epiphysis:* Phylogenetically represents a separate bone which in man has become fused to another bone, e.g., coracoid process of scapula.

(d) *Aberrant epiphysis:* These are not always present, e.g., Epiphysis at head of first metacarpal.

Q. How the bones are classified according to their structure?

Ans. (a) *Compact bone:* Dense and is developed in cortex of long bones. It is able to resist mechanical pressure.

(b) *Cancellous bone* (Spongy): Consists of meshwork of trabeculae (lamellae) within which are intercommunicating spaces, e.g., vertebral bodies, ribs, sternum.

Q. What are Sharpey's fibres?

Ans. These are the transverse fibres which hold the lamellae of the compact bone together and periosteum to the underlying bone.

Q. What are the different types of lamellae in a bone?

Ans. (a) *Circumferential lamellae:* Lie parallel to bony surface

(b) *Osteonic lamellae:* Concentric lamellae found around vascular canals of bone.

(c) *Interstitial lamellae:* Lie in space between osteons, *i.e.*, vascular canals.

Q. How the bones are classified according to their developmental origin?

Ans. (a) *Intramembranous (Dermal) bone:* Develops from direct transformation of condensed mesenchyme, e.g., bones of skull.

(b) *Intracartilaginous (Endochondral) bone:* Replaces a preformed cartilage model, e.g., bones of limb and thoracic cage.

(c) *Membranocartilaginous bone:* Develops partly in membrane and partly in cartilage, e.g., clavicle, mandible.

Q. What is Woff's law?

Ans. The mechanical stresses are directly proportional to the bone formation.

Q. What are centres of ossification?

Ans. These are certain constant points in a bone where the mineralization of connective tissue begins and the process of transformation spreads, until whole skeletal element is ossified.

Q. What is 'Law of ossification' for a long bone?

Ans. Where a bone has an epiphysis at either end, the epiphysis which is first to appear is last to join and the epiphysis which is last to appear is the first to join except fibula.

Q. What is the arterial supply of a long bone?

Ans. The arterial supply of a long bone is derived from four sources:

(a) *Nutrient artery:* It enters the shaft through nutrient foramen and runs obliquely in cortex and divides into ascending and descending branches in medullary cavity. Each branch inturn divides and redivides into parallel vessels, which run in metaphysis. These terminate by anastomising with epiphysial, metaphysial and periosteal arteries.
It supplies medullary cavity and inner 2/3 of cortex. The nutrient foramen is directed opposite to the growing end of bone.

(b) *Juxta-epiphysial (Metaphysial) arteries of Lexer:* These are derived from anastomosis around the joint. They pierce the metaphysis along line of attachment of joint capsule.

(c) *Epiphysial arteries:* Derived from periarticular vascular arcades found on non articular bony surface.

(d) *Periosteal arteries:* These ramify beneath periosteum and supply outer 1/3 of cortex.

Q. What are 'Sesamoid bones'? What are their characteristic features?

Ans.
1. These are bone nodules found embedded in tendons where they lie close to articular surface or turn around a bony surface and joint capsules.
2. These have no periosteum.
3. They are not always completely ossified and consist of fibrous tissue, cartilage and bone in varying proportion, e.g., in tendon of adductor pollicis and flexor pollicis brevis and in 70% cases in tendons anterior to metacarpophalangeal joint; patella; in tendon of flexor hallucis brevis, peroneus longus and tibialis posterior.

4. They ossify after birth
5. They have no Haversian system.

Q. What are the functions of sesamoid bones?

Ans. 1. Alter the direction of pull of muscle or improve the pull of the muscles.
2. To minimize friction.
3. To modify pressure.
4. Aids in maintaining the local circulation
5. Provide additional articular surface to a joint.

CARTILAGE

Q. What is cartilage and what are its characteristic features?

Ans. (a) It is a type of connective tissue, which has gel like ground substance known as matrix, in which are embedded cartilage cells (chondrocytes).
(b) The matrix is made up of mucopolysaccharide and contains elastic or collagen fibres.
(c) The cartilage is firm in consistency and has elasticity.
(d) It has no lymphatics or blood supply.
(e) It may become calcified.

Q. What are the different types of cartilage and their distribution?

Ans. (a) *Hyaline cartilage:* No fibres seen in matrix. Does not regenerate because chondrocytes cannot redivide. Present at articular surface of synovial joint bones, costal cartilage, bronchial cartilage.
(b) *Fibrocartilage:* Collagen fibres present in matrix. Present in intervertebral disc, discs in joints and on the articular surfaces of clavicle and mandible.
(c) *Elastic cartilage:* Elastic fibres present in cartilage, e.g., auditory tube, pinna and epiglottis.

Q. Name the cartilages which calcify.

Ans. (a) Hyaline cartilage
(b) Fibrocartilage

Q. How the different cartilages obtain their nourishment?

Ans. Fibrocartilage is supplied by blood vessels but hyaline and elastic cartilage have no capillaries and their cells are being nourished by diffusion of lymph.

ARTHROLOGY

Q. How the joints are classified according to their structure?

Ans. (a) *Fibrous joint:* Bones are joined together by fibrous tissue. These joints are immobile or permit only slight movement.

(b) *Cartilagenous joint:* Bones are joined together by cartilage.

(c) *Synovial joint:* Articular surfaces of bone are covered by articular (hyaline) cartilage and between articular surface is joint cavity, containing synovial fluid. These joints permit maximum degree of movement.

Q. What are the different types of fibrous joints?

Ans. (a) *Sutures:* Found in skull and are immobile. Sutural ligament is present between two bones, which is attached on outside to pericranium and endocranium (outer layer of duramater) on inside.

(b) *Syndesmosis:* Bones are connected by interosseous ligament, e.g., inferior tibiofibular joint.

(c) *Gomphosis:* Peg and socket type of joint, e.g., tooth in its socket.

Q. What are the characteristic features of synovial joint?

Ans. (a) Bony articular surfaces are covered with hyaline cartilage. It is insensitive to pain.

(b) Articular bones are connected by a fibrous capsule. The capsule has poor blood supply and heals very slowly. It is sensitive pain and stretch.

(c) Inner surface of capsule and all intra-articular structures which are not covered with cartilage are covered by synovial membrane, which secretes synovial fluid. It is highly vascular.

Q. What is the characteristic feature of synovial fluid?

Ans. It is presence of large amounts of mucopolysaccharide (hyaluronic acid) which gives it characteristic viscosity and it does not clot.

Q. What are the functions of synovial fluid?

Ans. 1. Lubrication of joint
2. Nourishes the articular cartilage.

Q. What are the different types of synovial joint?

Ans. (a) *Arthrodial (plane):* Flat surfaces are in contact. Only gliding movement is possible, e.g., intercarpal joints, intertarsal joints.

(b) *Hinge:* Movements take place around a transverse axis, e.g., Elbow joint between humerus and ulna.

(c) *Pivot:* A bony pivot like process moves within a ring. So movements are possible only around longitudinal axis through centre of pivot, e.g., Upper radio-ulnar joint and median atlantoaxial joint.

(d) *Condylar:* Two convex condyles (articular surface) moves within two concavities on opposite side. Movements occur mainly in transverse axis but partly in vertical axis (rotation), e.g., knee joint, temporo-mandibular joint, interphalangeal joints.

(e) *Ellipsoid:* Formed by a oval convex surface and an elliptical concavity, e.g., Radiocarpal joint (wrist joint), metacarpophalangeal joint. Movements possible are flexion, extension, abduction, adduction and circumduction. No rotation occurs around central axis.

(f) *Saddle:* Articular surfaces are both concavoconvex. Movements permitted are same as in condylar type with some rotational movements, e.g., carpometacarpal joint of thumb, ankle joint.

(g) *Ball and socket:* Articular surfaces are globular head which fit into a cup like cavity. Movements are possible in every direction around a common centre, e.g., hip joint, shoulder joint.

Q. What is a compound joint?

Ans. When more than two bone ends are enclosed with in a single capsule, the joint is known as compound, e.g., elbow joint has humeroulnar, humeroradial and superior radioulnar joint.

Q. What is a complex joint?

Ans. The joint cavity is divided completely or incompletely into two parts by intraarticular disc or fibrocartilage, e.g., temporomandibular joint, sternoclavicular joint and knee joint.

Q. How the joints are divided according to axis of movements?

Ans.

(a) *Multiaxial*	:	Ball and socket joints
(b) *Biaxial*	:	Ellipsoid and saddle joints
(c) *Uniaxial*	:	Hinge and pivot joints

Q. What are fatty pads? What is their importance?

Ans. These are found in some synovial joints, occupying spaces where bony surfaces are incongruous and are covered by synovial membrane, e.g.,

(a) Hip joint (Haversian fat pad),
(b) Talocalcaneonavicular joint,
(c) Infrapatellar fold and
(d) Alar folds of knee joints.

Q. What are different types of cartilaginous joints?

Ans. (a) *Primary (synchondroses):* The related bones are united by hyaline cartilage. They are immovable and the cartilage is replaced by bone with age, e.g., costochondral joints, joint between epiphysis and diaphysis of a growing long bone, between spenoid and temporal bones.

(b) *Secondary (symphysis):* These joints occur in median plane. The bone ends are covered by hyaline cartilage and are connected by a disc of fibrocartilage, e.g., manubrosternal joints, symphysis pubis, intervertebral joint between vertebral bodies. These do not disappear with age. Slight movement is possible.

Q. Why symphysis menti, joining two halves of mandible is not a true symphysis?

Ans. Because it disappears with age.

Q. What are the different intra-articular structures present in joints?

Ans. (a) *Cartilaginous structures*

1. *Articular disc*
   i. *Complete:* Mandibular joint and strenoclavicular joint
   ii. *Incomplete:* Acromioclavicular joint.
2. *Articular menisci:* Semilunar cartilages of knee joint.
3. *Labrum glenoidale:* Glenoid cavity of scapula and acetabulum.
4. *Ligaments traversing joints:* Bind articular surfaces, e.g., ligamentum teres of hip joint, cruciate ligaments of knee joint.

(b) *Muscle tendons*: These arise inside capsule of joint, e.g.,
   1. At shoulder joint, long head of biceps
   2. At knee joint, tendon of popliteus.

Q. What are the functions of intra-articular discs?

Ans. 1. They act as a buffer and absorb shock.
2. They strengthen the joint
3. They make the articulation between bony surfaces smooth and harmonious.

Q. What Hilton's law?

Ans. A joint is supplied by the same nerves which supply the muscles crossing the joint and skin over the joint. Therefore, in joint diseases, irritation of nerves cause reflex spasm of muscles and referred pain to the overlying skin.

MYOLOGY

Q. What are the distinguishing features of different types of muscle?

Ans.

	Features	Smooth muscle	Skeletal muscle	Cardiac muscle
(a)	Location	Found in viscera and blood vessels	Found attached to skeleton	Found in myocardium of heart

Contd.

Contd.

	Features	*Smooth muscle*	*Skeletal muscle*	*Cardiac muscle*
(b)	Nerve supply	Autonomic nerves, so they are involuntary	Somatic nerves, so they are involuntary	Autonomic nerves, so they are involuntary
(c)	Muscle fibre	Has no cross striations	Has cross striations	Has cross striations
		Each fibre is elongated, spindle shaped	Cylindrical cell	Muscle fibre show branches and anastomose with neighbouring fibres
		Single central nucleus	Multiple peripheral nuclei	Single central nucleus
(d)	Rhythmicity	Present	Absent	Present
(e)	Automaticity	Present	Absent	Present

Q. How the skeletal muscles are classified according to direction of muscle fibres?

Ans. (a) When the fasciculi (groups of muscle fibres) are parallel to line of pull, e.g.,

1. *Strap like:* Sternohyoid, sartorius.
2. *Fusiform:* Biceps
3. *Quadrilateral:* Thyrohyoid.

(b) When the fasciculi are oblique to line of pull e.g.,

1. *Triangular:* Temporalis, adductor longus.
2. *Pennate (Feather like):*
   - i. *Unipennate:* Extensor digitorum longus, flexor policis longus.
   - ii. *Bipennate:* Rectus femoris
   - iii. *Multipennate:* Deltoid, subscapularis
   - iv. *Circumpennate:* Tibialis anterior.

(c) When muscle fibres are arranged in a twisted manner, e.g., trapezius, pectoralis major.

Q. What is the nerve supply of skeletal muscle?

Ans. Supplied by somatic nerves.

1. *Motor fibres:* Has
   - (a) *Alpha efferents:* Myelinated anterior horn motor neurons, supply muscle fibres.
   - (b) *Gamma efferents:* Myelinated fibres, supply muscle spindle (sensory end organ of skeletal muscle).

(c) *Autonomic efferents:* Non myelinated, supply smooth muscle fibres of blood vessels.

2. *Sensory fibres:*
   (a) *Myelinated fibres:* Distributed to muscle spindle, tendon and fascia of the muscle.
   (b) *Non myelinated fibres:* Distribution not known.

Q. What is a 'motor unit'?

Ans. It is a functional subdivision of muscle. It includes a single alpha motor neuron together with muscle fibres which it innervates.

Q. What is myotome?

Ans A myotome is amount of muscle supplied by one segment of the spinal cord and muscles sharing a common primary action on a joint irrespective of their anatomical situation are supplied by the same segments.

Q. What are the features of muscles which receive 'Double innervation'?

Ans. Generally they are flexor muscles that receive nerve supply from the extensor compartment. These muscles develop in the extensor compartment of foetal limb but for functional reasons, come to lie in the flexor compartment of the adult limb, bringing its nerve supply with, *e.g.*,

(a) Lateral portion of brachialis (supplied by radial nerve).
(b) Short head of biceps femoris (By personal part of sciatic nerve).
(c) Brachioradialis (By radial nerve).

Q. What are bursae and where they are found?

Ans. Bursae are sacs of synovial membrane supported by dense irregular connective tissue.

They are found at the places where structures which move relative to each other are in tight apposition, e.g.,

(a) Between skin and bone *(Subcutaneous bursae)*
(b) Between muscle and bone, tendon or ligament *(Submuscular)*.
(c) Between fascia and bone *(Subfascial)*
(d) Between ligaments *(Interligamentous)*

(e) *Adventitious bursae:* Normally not present but develop over bony situations which are subject to much friction or pressure, e.g.,

1. *Tailor's ankle:* Above lateral malleolus a bursa appears in tailors, who sit in cross legged position, thus bringing this area in contact with table.
2. *Porter's shoulder:* In porters, between upper surface of clavicle and skin.
3. *Weaver's bottom:* Between gluteus maximus and ischial tuberosity.

Q. What is 'Aponeuroses'?

Ans. These are flat sheets of densely arranged collagen fibres associated with the attachment of muscle.

Q. What are the different types of muscles according to their action?

Ans. (a) *Prime movers:* These are active in initiation and maintenance of a particular movement.

(b) *Antagonists:* Muscles which oppose prime movers or initiate and maintain its converse.

(c) *Fixators:* Stabilize the position of a joint to provide a fixed base on which other muscles can act

(d) *Synergists:* These help the prime movers in bringing the movement. They eliminate the undesired actions when prime movers cross more than one joint.

CIRCULATORY SYSTEM

Q. What is the difference between arteries and veins?

Ans.

Features	*Arteries*	*Veins*
Thickness	Thick walled	Thin walled
Valves	Absent	Present
Lumen	Narrow	Larger
Fibromuscular tissue	More	Less
Elasticity	More	Less

Arteries carry oxygenated blood except pulmonary artery and veins carry deoxygenated blood except pulmonary veins.

Q. What are the differences between capillaries and sinusoids?

Ans.

Features	Capillary	Sinusoid
1. Lumen	Smaller, regular	Larger (upto 30 μ) irregular
2. Structure	*Endothelial lining:*	
	Continuous	May be incomplete; some phagocytic cells are present.
	Basal lamina:	
	Thicker and surround endothelial cells	Thinner
	Adventitial support:	
	Present	Absent
3. Location	Connect metaarterioles and venules	Connect arteriole with venule or venule with venule.

Q. Name the structures where fenestrated capillaries are present.

Ans. (a) Pancreas
(b) Intestine
(c) Renal glomeruli
(d) Endocrine glands

Q. Name the structures where continuous capillaries are present.

Ans. (a) Skin
(b) Muscles
(c) Fascia
(d) Brain

Q. What is the nerve supply of an artery?

Ans. The arteries are supplied by sympathetic nerves via nervi vasorum. These are vasoconstrictor. Few myelinated sympathetic fibres are also present, which carry pain sensation.

Q. Name the sites where sinusoids are present

Ans. (a) Suprarenal gland
(b) Carotid body
(c) Liver
(d) Spleen.

Q. What are 'Anastomosis'?

Ans. Arteries do not end always in capillaries, they unite with one another forming anastomosis.

Q. What are the different types of anastomosis?

Ans.
1. *Actual:* Arteries meet end to end, e.g., labial branches of facial arteries, intercostal arteries, uterine and ovarian arteries, arterial arcades in mesentery, arteries of greater and lesser curvatures of stomach.
2. *Potential:* Anastomosis is by terminal arterioles and given sufficient time the arterioles can dilate to take sufficient blood, e.g., coronary arteries, cortical arteries of cerebral hemispheres, anastomoses around joints of extremities.

Q. What are the functions of anastomosis?

Ans. (a) Equalization of pressure over territories which they connect.

(b) Provide collateral circulation when a vessel is interrupted.

Q. What are 'End arteries'? What is their importance?

Ans. These are arteries which have no anastomoses with their neighbours, e.g., Central artery of retina, arteries of spleen, liver, kidneys, metaphyses of long bones, medullary branches of the central nervous system, coronary arteries.

Importance: If an end artery is occluded, necrosis (death) of tissue takes place in area supplied by the vessel.

Q. What are 'Arteriovenous shunts'?

Ans. These are vessels of communication between arteries and veins and when open, they bypass the capillaries, e.g., in skin of nose, lips and external ear, mucous membrane of alimentary canal, thyroid gland, palmar skin.

Q. What are the functions of arteriovenous shunts?

Ans.
1. Regulate the regional blood flow
2. Regulate blood pressure
3. Pressor reception
4. Regulation of the temperature.

LYMPHATIC SYSTEM

Q. What are the components of lymphatic system?

Ans (a) *Lymph vessels:* Formed by lymph capillaries.

(b) *Peripheral lymphoid tissue:* Spleen, epithelio-lymphoid system, lymph nodes and lymph nodules.

(c) *Central lymphoid tissue:* Bone marrow and thymus.

(d) *Lymphocytes:* Circulating in vessels.

Q. How the lymph capillaries differ from blood capillaries?

Ans. Lymph capillaries have

(a) Bigger lumen

(b) Lumen is less regular

(c) Permeable to bigger molecules

(d) Form pathways for absorption of colloid from tissue spaces

Q. Name the sites were lymph capillaries are absent.

Ans. (a) Epidermis

(b) Hair

(c) Nails

(d) Cornea

(e) Articular cartilage

(f) Splenic pulp

(g) Spinal cord

(h) Brain and

(i) Bone marrow

Q. What is the structure of lymph trunk?

Ans. It consists of three coats:

(a) *Tunica adventitia:* Composed mainly of fibrous tissue and some smooth muscle fibres

(b) *Tunica media:* Consists of smooth muscles cells, fibres of which are arranged circularly and separated from one another by fibrous tissue.

(c) *Tunica intima:* Consist of endothelial cells and fibrous tissue.

They possess more number of valves than small veins. The valve consists of reduplicated endothelium and lumen of lymph vessel immediately proximal to valve is expanded into a *sinus*, which gives the vessel a *beaded appearance*.

Q. What are the factors which favour the propulsion of lymph from tissue spaces towards lymph nodes and venous blood stream?

Ans. (a) In tissue spaces, filtration pressure generated by filtration of fluid from blood capillaries.
(b) Concentration of surrounding muscles compressing lymph vessels
(c) Pulsation of artery near lymph vessels
(d) Respiratory movements
(e) Negative pressure in brachiocephalic veins
(f) Contraction of smooth muscle of vessel.

Q. What is the function of lymph capillaries?

Ans Lymph capillaries are concerned with the absorption of fluid from tissue spaces.

Q. What is structure of lymph node?

Ans. *Grossly:*

These are oval bodies situated in the course of lymph vessels. The blood vessels enter and leave node at the hilus. A lymph node has a *cortex* into which afferent vessels drain and a *medulla* from which efferent vessels arise.

Microscopic:

(a) *Capsule and trabeculae:* Composed of collagen fibres, fibroblasts and elastic fibres.
(b) *Reticulum:* Fibrocellular and forms a meshwork within spaces outlined by capsule and trabeculae. In medulla, fewer cells in loose reticulum are present. Such parts allow rapid passage of lymph and are termed *lymph sinuses*. Reticular fibres are thin collagen fibres, ensheathed by fixed macrophages in an amorphous matrix. Reticular cells lining lymph sinuses are termed as *littoral cells*.

Majority of cells are lymphocytes with some macrophages. In cortex, cells are densely packed to form *lymphatic follicles*. The central part of follicle has a *germinal centre*, which consists of large cells. In medulla, cells are loosely packed.

The outer part of cortex has B-lymphocytes and inner part has T-lymphocytes. The medulla has mature B-lymphocytes, plasma cells and macrophages.

Q. What is epithelio-lymphoid system and where it is found?

Ans. These are collections of lymphoid tissue found under the epithelium.

These are found in Peyer's patches in intestine, appendix, pharyngeal tonsil, palatine and lingual tonsil.

Q. What are the different type of cells in reticulo-endothelial system?

Ans. These cells are concerned with phagocytosis.

(a) Pericytes (Rouget cells) in capillaries
(b) Dust cells in lungs
(c) Macrophages in connective tissue, bone marrow and suprarenal gland
(d) Reticular cells in spleen and lymphoid tissue
(e) Monocytes in blood
(f) Kupffer cells in liver
(g) Microglia in nervous system.

Q. What are the functions of a lymph node?

Ans. (a) Act as a filter for lymph. Thus, foreign particles are prevented from entering the blood stream.
(b) macrophages in sinuses engulf foreign particles.
(c) Trapping of antigens by phagocytes
(d) Mature B and T lymphocytes are produced in the lymph node.
(e) Provides interaction between antigen laden phagocytes and lymphoid tissue with mounting of both cellular and humoral immune response.
(f) Provides portal of entry for blood borne lymphocytes back into lymphatic channels.

NERVOUS SYSTEM

Q. What are the subdivisions of nervous system?

Ans. (a) *Central nervous system:* Includes brain and spinal cord.
(b) *Peripheral nervous system:* Divides into:
1. *Cerebrospinal nervous system:* Includes 12 pairs of cranial nerves and 31 pair of spinal nerves.

2. *Peripheral autonomic nervous system:* Includes sympathetic and parasympathetic nervous system.

Q. What are the cell types forming nervous tissue?

Ans. (a) *Neurons (Nerve cells):* Excitable cells.

(b) *Neuroglia:* Non excitable cells, forming connective tissue of the nervous system.

Q. What is the function of neurons?

Ans. Reception, transmission, integration and transformation of impulses.

Q. What is the histological structure of a neuron?

Ans. Each neuron consists of:

(a) *Cell body (Perikaryon):* Mass of cytoplasm with a diploid núcleus and bound by a membrane. The cytoplasm contains basophilic Nissl bodies. Nissl body is made of ribonucleic acid and is concerned with the protein synthesis.

(b) *Neurites:* Extensions from periphery of cell body. They are of two types:

1. *Dendrites:* Conduct impulses towards cell body. May branch to form a dendritic tree.
2. *Axon:* Conduct impulses away from cell body. Begins at *axon hillock* and terminate by dividing into axon terminals *(telodendria)*.

Q. What are the different types of neurons?

Ans. (a) *Unipolar:* Single extension from cell body, e.g., mesencephalic nucleus of fifth cranial nerve.

(b) *Bipolar:* Extension at each end of the cell body, e.g., Retinal bipolar cells, olfactory neuroepithelium and ganglion of 8th cranial nerve.

(c) *Multipolar:* Several extensions from cell body, e.g., Most cells of brain and spinal cord.

(d) *Pseudo-unipolar:* Usually have one process arising are pole óf cell body but actually two extensions emerge at same pole, e.g., dorsal root ganglion of spinal cord.

Q. What are Amacrine cells?

Ans. These are small neurons present in retina, olfactory bulb which lack an obvious axon and permit conduction in either direction.

Q. What are the different types of neurons in brain?

Ans. (a) *Stellate cells:* Dendrites extend in all directions from cell body.

(b) *Pyramidal cells:* Cell body is conical in shape and dendrites extend from angles of cone or pyramid.

(c) *Fusiform cells:* Spindle shaped dendrites emerge at both ends.

(d) *Glomerular cells:* Dendrites at their tip are highly coiled.

Q. What is a 'Synapse'?

Ans. Sites of junction between two neurons which permit interneuronal transmission of impulses. the presynaptic and postsynaptic process are separated by a small gap, *synaptic cleft.*

Q. What are the different types of synapse?

Ans. Depending on the type of neuronal process involved and direction of transmission synapses are classified into:

(a) *Axodendritic:* Commonest

(b) Axosomatic

(c) Dendrosomatic

(d) Dendroxaonic

(e) Dendrodendritic and

(f) Axoaxonic.

Q. How transmission occurs across the synapse?

Ans. Due to the release of transmitters (Neurochemicals) released into the synaptic cleft by presynaptic process, which cause the stimulation or inhibition of post-synaptic process.

Q. What are the different types of synapse?

Ans. 1. *Excitatory synapse:* Neurotransmitters released causes stimulation of post synaptic neuron.

2. *Inhibitory synapse:* Neurotransmitter released causes inhibition of post synaptic neuron.

3. *Reciprocal synapses:* Transmission between two processes occurs in either direction by staggered synaptic zones on each side of synaptic cleft.

Q. What are different types of neuroglial cells in brain and spinal cord?

Ans. (a) *Macroglia:* Larger cells, develop from neural plate. They are of following types:

1. *Astrocytes:* Have a small cell body with dendrite like extensions.
2. *Oligodendrocytes:* They have fewer cell processes.
3. *Pituicytes:* In posterior pituitary
4. *Muller cells:* In retina.
5. *Ependymal cells:* Line the ventricles of brain and central canal of spinal cord
6. *Bergman cells:* In cerebellum.

(b) *Microglia:* Smallest glial cells. They have fine dendritic processes and flattened outlines. Develop from mesodermal tissue surrounding nervous system.

Q. What are the functions of glial cells?

Ans. 1. Act as mechanical support for nervous system.
2. Act as insulators, separating neurons and their processes from each other. They prevent impulses from spreading in unwanted directions due to their non conducting nature.
3. Act defensively by phagocytosing foreign material and cell debris.
4. Help in regulating biochemical environment of neurons.
5. Oligodendrocytes form myelin sheath in central nervous system.
6. Ependymal cells take part in secretion, transport and uptake of cerebrospinal fluid.
7. By proliferation, glial çells repair, by filling the gaps left by dead or degenerating neurons.
8. They take up, store and metabolise the neurotransmitters.

Q. What are the different types of fibres in peripheral nerve?

Ans. Depending on diameter and rate of impulse conduction fibres in peripheral nerve are of three types:

(a) *Type A:* Subdivided into:

1. Sensory (Afferent) fibres
2. Motor (Efferent) fibres

(b) *Type B:* Preganglonic autonomic fibres

(c) *Type C:* Nonmyelinated, post ganglionic autonomic fibres

Q. What are the factors on which conduction in myelinated fibres depend?

Ans. (a) Diameter of axon

(b) Thickness of myelin sheath

(c) Internodal distance between nodes of Ranvier

(d) Area and character of axonal membrane.

Q. What are the non-nervous cells present in peripheral nervous system?

Ans. (a) *Capsular cells:* Present around cell body of sensory and autonomic ganglia.

(b) *Schwann cells:* Present around axons of peripheral nerves and form myelin sheath.

Q. What is the composition of myelin?

Ans. Myelin contains lipid and basic proteins but has less proteins than cell membrane.

Q. What are 'Incisures of Schmidt-Lanterman'?

Ans. These are oblique clefts in the myelin and provide conduction channels for metabolities into depths of myelin sheath and axon.

Q. What is the characteristic feature of distribution of sympathetic and parasympathetic nervous system?

Ans. All parts of body, whether somatic or visceral, receive a sympathetic supply.

But the parasympathetic supply has no somatic distribution but is wholly visceral, but does not innervate all viscera (e.g., suprarenal glands and gonads, which have only a sympathetic supply).

Q. What is the origin of autonomic nervous system outflow?

Ans. Sympathetic outflow emerges at T_1 to L_2 segments of spinal cord.

Parasympathetic outflow emerges from brain via 3rd, 7th, 9th and 10th cranial nerves and from S_{2-4} segments of spinal cord.

Q. To which gland the secretomotor nerves are sympathetic?

Ans. Sweat glands.

Q. Which cranial nerves contribute to the cranial parasympathetic outflow?

Ans. Preganglionic fibres from third, seventh, ninth and tenth cranial nerves.

Q. What is the neurotransmitter of autonomic nervous system?

Ans. Noradrenaline is neurotransmitter of sympathetic system except at nerves ending for sweat gland and blood vessels of muscles, where neurotransmitter is acetylcholine.

Acetylcholine is neurotransmitter of parasympathetic system.

Upper Limb

BONES OF UPPER LIMB

CLAVICLE

Q. What are the characteristic features of clavicle?

Ans. 1. It is a long bone which lies horizontally in body.
2. It has no medullary cavity.
3. It is subcutaneous throughout.
4. It is the first bone to ossify in body of fetus.
5. Only long bone that ossifies in membrane except sternal and acromial end.
6. It is the only long bone which ossifies from two primary centres.
7. It is the most commonly fractured bone in body.

Q. How will you determine the side to which clavicle belongs?

Ans. 1. It was two ends, lateral and medial. Lateral end is flat and medial end is large and quadrilateral.
2. Shaft is convex forwards in medial 2/3 and concave forwards in lateral 1/3.
3. Inferior surface is grooved longitudinally in middle 1/3.

Q. What is the nutrient artery supplying clavicle?

Ans. Nutrient branch from suprascapular artery.

Q. What are the muscles attached to the medial part of clavicle?

Ans. a. Clavicular part of pectoralis major: From anterior surface of medial half.
b. Clavicular head of sternocleidomastoid: From upper surface of medial part.
c. Lateral part of sternohyoid: Posterior surface of medial end.

Q. What are the functions of clavicle?

Ans. (a) Transmits force from upper limb to axial skeleton.
(b) Provides attachment to muscles.
(c) Acts as a strut holding arm free from trunk.

Q. Name the structures attached to the edges of groove for subclavius.

Ans. Clavipectoral fascia.

Q. To which structure the medial end of clavicle articulates?

Ans. a. Manubrium sterni
b. First costal cartilage

Q. At which site the clavicle fracture occurs commonly?

Ans. At junction of middle and outer third, which is the weakest point.

SCAPULA

Q. What is the extent and position of scapula?

Ans. 1. It lies on posterolateral aspect of chest wall.
2. It extends from II to VII rib.

Q. How will you determine side to which scapula belongs?

Ans. 1. Lateral angle is large and has a glenoid cavity.
2. Lateral thickest border runs from glenoid cavity above to the inferior angle below.
3. Dorsal surface is convex and is divided into supraspinatus and infraspinatus fossa by triangular spine.
4. Costal surface is concave.

Q. Name the structures passing above and below suprascapular notch.

Ans. The suprascapular notch is converted into a foramen by the suprascapular ligament.
The suprascapular artery passes above the ligament and suprascapular nerve below the ligament.

Q. Name the structures attached to Acromion.

Ans. (a) *Trapezius:* Inserted on its medial border
(b) *Deltoid:* Originates from lateral margin, tip and upper surface.
(c) *Coracoacromial ligament:* Attached to apex of acromion.

Q. What are the structures attached to coracoid process?

Ans. *Muscles:*
(a) *Short head of biceps:* Origin from tip of coracoid process.
(b) *Coracobrachialis:* Origin from tip of coracoid process.
(c) *Pectoralis minor:* Insertion on medial border and superior surface.

Ligaments:
(a) *Coracoacromial ligament:* To lateral border.
(b) *Coracoclavicular ligament: Conoid part* to knuckle of process. *Trapezoid part* to ridge between pectoralis minor and coraco-acromial ligament.
(c) *Coracohumeral ligament:* To root of coracoid process.

Q. Name the muscles inserting on the medial border of scapula?

Ans. *On costal surface*: Insertion of two digitations of serratus anterior.
On dorsal surface: Insertion of
(a) *Levator scapulae:* Above root of spine
(b) *Rhomboideus minor:* Opposite the root
(c) *Rhomboideus major:* Below the root.

Q. Which muscle originates from supraglenoid tubercle?

Ans. Long head of biceps.

Q. Which muscle originates from infraglenoid tubercle?

Ans. Long head of triceps.

Q. How many ossification centres are present in scapula?

Ans. Eight.

HUMERUS

Q. How will you determine the side to which the humerus belongs?

Ans. 1. Upper end is rounded and forms the head. Lower end is flattened from before backwards.
2. Head is directed medially and backwards.
3. Lesser tubercle projects from front of upper end.
4. The anterior aspect of upper end shows a vertical groove called intertubercular sulcus.

Q. What is the anatomical position of the humerus in body?

Ans. 1. Head is directed medially, upwards and backwards.
2. Medical epicondyle is directed medially and slightly backwards.

Q. What are contents of intertubercular sulcus (Bicipital groove)?

Ans. 1. Tendon of long head of biceps.
2. Synovial sheath of the tendon.
3. Ascending branch of anterior circumflex humeral artery.

Q. What are the structures attached to intertubercular sulcus?

Ans. 1. *To medial lip:* Teres major, insertion.
2. *To floor:* Latissimus dorsi, insertion.
3. *To lateral lip:* Pectoralis major, insertion.

Q. How the tendon of pectoralis major is inserted?

Ans. It is inserted by a bilaminar tendon on the lateral lip of bicipital groove, the two laminae are continuous with each other inferiorly.

Q. What are the muscles inserting on greater tubercle?

Ans. (a) *Supraspinatus:* On upper impression,
(b) *Infraspinatus:* On middle impression,
(c) *Teres minor:* On lower impression.

Q. Which muscle is inserted into lesser tubercle?

Ans. Supscapularis

Q. What is the 'anatomical neck' and 'surgical neck' of humerus?

Ans. *Anatomical neck*: Surrounds the margin of head. Provides attachment to capsular ligament which is deficient inferiorily on medial side.

Surgical neck: Lies at upper end of shaft, below the epiphyseal line. It is a common site for fracture.

Q. What are the structures related to surgical neck of humerus?

Ans. 1. Axillary nerve
2. Anterior and posterior circumflex humeral vessels.

Q. Name the structures related to radial groove of shaft of humerus.

Ans. 1. Radial nerve and
2. Profunda brachii vessels.

Q. Which muscle originates from medial supracondylar ridge?

Ans. Pronator teres, from lower end of medial supracondylar ridge.

Q. Which muscle originates from lateral supracondylar ridge?

Ans. 1. Brachioradialis: From upper two thirds,
2. Extensor carpi radialis longus: From lower one third.

Q. Which muscles arise from lateral epicondyle of humerus (common extensor origin)?

Ans. a. Extensor carpi radialis brevis
b. Extensor digitorum
c. Extensor digiti minimi
d. Extensor carpi ulnaris

Q. Which muscles also arise from lateral epicondyle of humerus except from common extensor origin?

Ans. a. Anconeus
b. Supinator

Q. What is angle of 'Humeral torsion'?

Ans. It is an angle formed by superimposition of long axes of upper and low articular surfaces of humerus.

It is about 164 degrees.
It is greater in man and in adults.

Q. What are fossae present in lower end of humerus?

Ans. 1. *Olecranon fossa:* Posteriorly, just above trochlea. Accommodates olecranon process in extended elbow.
2. *Radial fossa:* Anteriorly, above capitulum. Accommodates radial head in flexed elbow.
3. *Coronoid fossa:* Anteriorly, above trohlea. Accommodates coronoid process of ulna in flexed elbow.

Q. Why the fracture of humerus at junction of upper and middle third leads to delayed union?

Ans. Because of poor blood supply at the junction.

Q. Which nerve is most commonly involved in the supracondylar fracture of the humerus?

Ans. Median nerve.

Q. What are the ossification centres for lower end of humerus and at what age they appear?

Ans. 1. Capitulum: First year
2. Medial epicondyle: Fifth year
3. Medial part of trochlea: Ninth year
4. Lateral epicondyle: Twelfth year

Medial epicondyle fuses with shaft at 20th year and others fuse together to form a single epiphysis, which fuses with shaft at 15 years of age.

RADIUS AND ULNA

Q. How will you determine the side to which the radius belongs?

Ans. *Upper end:* Narrow and has a disc shaped head
Lower end: Wide, smooth anteriorly and ridges and grooves on posterior aspect.
Shaft: Convex laterally and concave forwards in lower part. Medial border is sharp.

Q. Where the biceps brachii is inserted?

Ans. Into rough posterior part of radial tuberosity.

Q. What structures are related to posterior aspect of lower end of radius?

Ans. 1. The groove behind medial part of lower end lodges tendons of extensor digitorum and extensor indicis.
2. The oblique groove medial to dorsal tubercle lodges tendon of extensor pollicis longus
3. The groove lateral to dorsal tubercle lodges tendons of extensor carpi radialis longus and brevis
4. The lateral aspect is crossed by tendons of abductor pollicis longus and extensor pollicis brevis.

Q. How will you determine the side to which ulna belongs?

Ans. 1. Upper end is hook like, with its concavity directed forwards.
2. Lateral border of shaft is sharp.

Q. Name the structures attached to medial surface of olecranon process.

Ans. *Upper part:*
1. Origin of ulnar head of flexor carpi ulnaris.
2. Posterior and oblique bands of ulnar collateral ligaments.

Lower part:
Upper fibres of flexor digitorum profundus.

Q. Name the structures attached to anterior surface of coronoid process.

Ans. *Whole of surface*: Insertion to brachialis.
Medial margin:
(a) Ulnar head of pronator teres,
(b) Ulnar head of flexor pollicis longus,
(c) Humeroulnar head of flexor digitorum superficialis,
(d) Anterior and oblique bands of ulnar collateral ligament.

Q. Name the muscles arising from aponeurosis of posterior border of shaft of ulna.

Ans. 1. Flexor digitorum profundus,
2. Flexor carpi ulnaris and
3. Extensor carpi ulnaris.

Q. What are the muscles arising from the lateral part of the posterior surface?

Ans. From above downwords,

(a) Abductor pollicis longus
(b) Extensor pollicis longus
(c) Extensor indicis

Q. What is Colle's fracture?

Ans. In adults, fall on the out stretched hand causes fracture of radius about one inch proximal to wrist joint and distal fragment is impacted dorsally and laterally.

Q. What is 'Students' elbow or 'Miner's elbow?

Ans. Inflammation of subcutaneous bursa present over olecranon due to repeated trauma. Commonly seen in miners and students.

BONES OF HAND

Q. Name the carpal bones.

Ans. *Proximal row:* Contains from lateral to medial side

1. Scaphoid,
2. Lunate,
3. Triquetral and
4. Pisiform

Distal row: Contains from lateral to medial side

1. Trapezium,
2. Trapezoid.
3. Capitate and
4. Hammate.

Q. Name the structures attached to tubercle of scaphoid.

Ans. 1. Abductor pollicis brevis and
2. Flexor retinaculum.

Q. Name the structures attached to pisiform.

Ans. 1. Flexor carpi ulnaris,
2. Abductor digiti minimi,
3. Flexor retinaculum and
4. Extensor retinaculum.

Q. Name the site of insertion of various muscles of thumb.

Ans. a. *Flexor pollicis longus:* Volar surface of base of distal phalanx

b. *Extensor pollicis longus:* Base of distal phalanx of thumb

c. *Extensor pollicis brevis:* Dorsal surface of base of proximal phalanx

d. *Abductor pollicis longus:* Base of first metacarpal

e. *Abductor pollicis, flexor pollicis brevis and abductor pollicis brevis:* Base of proximal phalanx of thumb

f. *Opponens pollicis:* Shaft of Ist metacarpal

g. *First palmar interossei:* Base of proximal phalanx.

Q. Name the muscles attached to middle phalanx.

Ans. 1. *Flexor digitorum superficialis:* Inserted on sides of shaft.

2. *Extensor digitorum:* Central slip inserted on dorsal surface of base.

Q. Name the structures attached to base of proximal phalanx.

Ans. Insertion of lumbricals and interossei.

In thumb, insertion of

1. *On lateral side:* Abductor pollicis brevis and flexor pollicis brevis.
2. *On medial side:* Abductor pollicis and first palmar interosseous.
3. *On dorsal surface:* Extensor pollicis brevis.

In little finger,

On medial side: Insertion of abductor digiti minimi and flexor digiti minimi.

Q. What are the sesamoid bones found in upper limb?

Ans. (a) *Pisiform:* Sesamoid bone within tendon of flexor carpi ulnaris.

(b) Two sesamoid bones on head of first metacarpal bone.

(c) In capsule of interphalangeal joint of thumb.

(d) On ulnar side of capsule of metacarpophalangeal joint of little finger.

JOINTS OF UPPER LIMB

SHOULDER JOINT

Q. What type of joint shoulder joint is?

Ans. Ball and socket variety of synovial joint.

Q. What are the articular surfaces of shoulder joint?

Ans. Glenoid cavity of scapula and head of humerus.

Q. Name the ligaments of shoulder joint?

Ans.
1. Capsular ligament.
2. Coracohumeral ligament.
3. Transverse humeral ligament.
4. Glenoidal labrum.

Q. What is the arterial supply of shoulder joint?

Ans.
1. Anterior circumflex humeral artery.
2. Posterior circumflex humeral artery.
3. Suprascapular artery and
4. Subscapular artery.

Q. What are the movements possible at shoulder joint? Name also the main muscle producing these movement?

Ans.
1. *Flexion:*
   (a) Clavicular head of pectoralis major
   (b) Anterior fibres of deltoid.
   (c) Coracobrachialis
   (d) Short head of biceps
2. *Extension:*
   (a) Sternocostal head to pectoralis major
   (b) Posterior fibres of deltoid
   (c) Latissimus dorsi
   (d) Teres major.
3. *Adduction:*
   (a) Pectoralis major
   (b) Latissimus dorsi
   (c) Subscapularis
   (d) Teres major.
4. *Abduction:*
   (a) Middle fibres of deltoid
   (b) Supraspinatus

5. *Medial rotation:*
   (a) Pectoralis major
   (b) Anterior fibres of deltoid
   (c) Latissimus dorsi
   (d) Teres major
   (e) Subscapularis.
6. *Lateral rotation:*
   (a) Posterior fibres of deltoid
   (b) Infraspinatus
   (c) Teres minor.
7. *Circumduction:* Combination of different movements.

Q. Name the bursa around shoulder joint.

Ans. (a) Subacromial bursa
(b) Subscapularis bursa
(c) Infraspinatus bursa
(d) Bursa related to muscles around shoulder joint e.g., teres major, long head of triceps, coracobrachialis.

Q. (a) Why shoulder joint is a week joint?
(b) How its stability is increased?

Ans. (a) 1. The glenoid cavity is shallow and small.
2. Head of humerus is larger than glenoid cavity.
(b) 1. By musculotendinous cuff of shoulder.
2. Coracoacromial arch.
3. Glenoidal labrum, which deepens the glenoid cavity and articular cartilage lining it.
4. Long muscles of shoulder, e.g., deltoid, long head of triceps, lattissimus dorsi and teres major.

Q. What is 'Rotator cuff' or 'Musculotendinous cuff'?

Ans. It is a fibrous sheath of tendons of short muscles of shoulder which cover all except inferior aspects of shoulder joint. The muscles are supraspinatus (superiorly) subscapularis (anteriorly), infraspinatus and teres minor (posteriorly).
The cuff gives strength to the capsule of shoulder joint.

Q. Which tendon is most commonly injured in rotator cuff lesions?

Ans. Supraspinatus.

Q. Why the dislocation of the shoulder joint occurs inferiorly?

Ans. Because the inferior aspect is unprotected by musculotendinous cuff.

Q. What is the clinical importance of shoulder tip pain?

Ans. Irritation of undersurface of diaphragm from surrounding pathology causes *referred pain* in the shoulder, because the phrenic nerve and supraclavicular nerves have similar root values ($C_{3,4}$).
Pain in the left shoulder tip due to irritation by splenic rupture.
Pain in the right shoulder, due to subphrenic abscess.
Acute pancreatitis and gas under the diaphragm due to perforation of peptic ulcer causes referred pain in the either of the shoulder tip.

SHOULDER GIRDLE

Q. What are the joints of shoulder girdle?

Ans. (a) Sternoclavicular joint
(b) Acromioclavicular joint.

Q. What type of joints are joints of shoulder girdle?

Ans. (a) *Sternoclavicular joint:* Saddle variety of synovial joint.
(b) *Acromioclavicular joint:* Plane variety of synovial joint.

Q. What is the characteristic feature of acromioclavicular joint?

Ans. It is partially divided by an incomplete fibrocartilage articular disc, which is perforated in the centre.

Q. Name the ligaments forming acromioclavicular joint?

Ans. a. Coracoclavicular ligament: Main ligament
b. Coracoacromial ligament

Q. What are the movements produced at the shoulder girdle?

Ans.

1. *Elevation of scapula:*
   (a) By upper fibres of trapezius and
   (b) Levator scapulae. Eg., shurgging of shoulders.
2. *Depression of scapula:* By
   (a) Lower fibres of serratus anterior,
   (b) Pectoralis minor
   (c) Levator scapulae and rhomboids also assist.
3. *Protraction of the scapula:* By
   (a) Serratus anterior and
   (b) Pectoralis minor. Eg., Punching movements.
4. *Retraction of scapulaL:* By
   (a) Rhomboids and
   (b) Middle fibres of trapezius.
5. *Forward rotation of scapula around chest wall:* In overhead abduction of shoulder by
   (a) Upper fibres of trapezius and
   (b) Lower fibres of serratus anterior.
6. *Backward rotation of scapula:* By
   (a) Levator scapulae and
   (b) Rhomboids.

Q. What is the function of shoulder girdle?

Ans. It suspends the upper limb to axial skeleton.

ELBOW JOINT

Q. What type of joint elbow joint is?

Ans. Hinge variety of synovial joint.

Q. What are the surfaces of elbow joint?

Ans. *From above:* Capitulum and trochlea of humerus
From below:
(a) Capitulum articulates with upper surface of head of radius
(b) Trochlear notch of ulna articulates with trochlea of humerus.

Q. Name the ligaments of elbow joint.

Ans. (a) Capsular ligament.
(b) Anterior ligament.
(c) Posterior ligament.
(d) Ulnar collateral ligament.
(e) Radial Collateral ligament.

Q. What are the movements of elbow joint? Name the muscles producing these movements.

Ans. *Flexion:* By
(a) Brachialis,
(b) Biceps and
(c) Brachioradialis.
Extension: By
(a) Triceps and
(b) Anconeus.

Q. How will you clinically test for dislocation of elbow joint?

Ans. Normally, in semiflexed position, olecranon and two humeral epicondyles form a equilateral triangle. In dislocation of elbow, this relationship is disturbed.

Q. What is 'Tennis Elbow'?

Ans. It is due to the partial tear of the common origin of the superficial extensor muscles of forearm.

Q. What is 'Golfer's Elbow'?

Ans. It is due to partial tear of the common origin of the superficial flexor muscles of forearm.

Q. What is student's/miner's elbow?

Ans. Repeated pressure over olecranon process leading to inflammation of olecranon bursa.

CUBITAL FOSSA

Q. What is cubital fossa?

Ans. It is a triangular hollow in front of elbow.

Q. What are the boundaries of cubital fossa?

Ans. *Laterally:* Medial border of brachioradialis.
Medially: Lateral border of pronator teres.

Base: By an imaginary line joining two epicondyles of the humerus.

Apex: By meeting point of lateral and medial boundaries.

Floor: By

(i) Brachialis and
(ii) Supinator.

Roof:

(i) Skin,
(ii) Superficial fascia
(iii) Deep fascia and
(iv) Bicipital aponeurosis.

Q. What are the contents of cubital fossa?

Ans. 1. Median nerve.
2. Termination of brachial artery.
3. Tendon of biceps with bicipital aponeurosis.
4. Radial nerve.

Q. Name the structures lying in superficial fascia of cubital fossa.

Ans. 1. Median cubital vein
2. Lateral cutaneous nerve of forearm
3. Medial cutaneous nerve of forearm.

Q. What is the clinical importance of median cubital vein?

Ans. It is the vein of choice for intravenous injections because it is fixed by perforator, so it does not slip away from needle.

Q. What is carrying angle?

Ans. It is the angle between long axis of arm with long axis of forearm, when forearm is extended and supinated. It disappears in full flexion of elbow and in pronation. It is about 170°.

Q. What are the factors responsible for carrying angle?

Ans. (a) Medial flange of trochlea is larger than lateral flange and projects downward to a lower level. As a result lower edge of trochlea passes downwards and medially.

(b) Superior articular surface of coronoid process of ulna is oblique.

Q. What is the importance and sex differences in carrying angle?

Ans. *Importance:*

1. It allows the arm to swing clearly away from the body.
2. The forearm comes in line with long axis of arm in midprone position in which the hand is mostly used.

Sex differences: Greater in females because of wider pelvis.

RADIO-ULNAR JOINTS

Q. What type of joint radioulnar joints are?

Ans. (a) *Superior radioulnar joint:* Pivot type of synovial joint.

(b) *Inferior radioulnar joint:* Pivot type of synovial joint.

(c) *Middle radioulnar joint:* Syndesmoses type of fibrous joint.

Q. What are the functions of interosseous membrane of middle radioulnar joint?

Ans. 1. Attachment to muscles,

2. Transmits weight of hand from radius to ulna.

Q. What is pronation and supination?

Ans. These are rotatory movements of forearm with hand around a vertical axis in semiflexed position.

In pronation, palm faces downwards

In supination, palm faces upwards.

Q. What is the axis of pronation and supination?

Ans. Vertical axis passing superiorly, through centre of head of radius and inferiorly, through apex of articular disc when ulna is fixed or through any fixed finger when ulna is free to move.

Q. Name the muscles producing pronation and supination.

Ans. (a) *Pronation:*

Principal muscles: Pronator teres, Pronator quadratus.

Accessory muscles: Flexor carpi radialis, Palmaris longus.

(b) *Supination:* Supinator and Biceps brachii.

WRIST JOINT

Q. What type of joint wrist joint is?

Ans. Ellipsoid variety of synovial joint.

Q. What are the articular surfaces of wrist joint?

Ans. *From above:*

(a) *Radius:* Inferior surface of lower end.

(b) Triangular articular disc of inferior radioulnar joint.

From below: Carpal bones: Scaphoid, Lunate and Triquetral.

Q. Name of the ligaments of wrist joint.

Ans. (a) Capsular ligament

(b) Anterior radiocarpal and ulnocarpal

(c) Posterior radiocarpal ligament

(d) Radial collateral ligament

(e) Ulnar collateral ligament.

Q. At which joint, movements of wrist take place?

Ans. (a) *Radiocarpal joint:* Mainly extension and adduction.

(b) *Midcarpal joint:* Mainly flexion and abduction.

Q. Name the muscles producing abduction and adduction at wrist joint.

Ans. *Abduction:*

(a) Flexor carpi radialis,

(b) Extensor carpi radialis longus and brevis,

(c) Extensor pollicis brevis and

(d) Abductor pollicis longus.

Adduction:

(a) Flexor carpi ulnaris and

(b) Extensor carpi ulnaris.

Q. Why the range of adduction is greater than abduction?

Ans. Because of longer styloid process of radius, which limits the abduction.

Q. What are the boundaries of 'Anatomical Snuffbox'?

Ans. It is depression on lateral side of wrist, when the thumb is extended.

Anterior:

(i) Abductor pollicis longus and

(ii) Extensor pollicis brevis.

Posterior: Extensor pollicis longus.

Pulsations of the radial artery can be felt in the floor of the depression against the scaphoid and trapezium and in the proximal part, styloid process of the radius and base of the thumb metacarpal distally.

JOINTS OF HAND

Q. What type of joint first carpometacarpal joint is?

Ans. Saddle variety of synovial joint.

Q. What is characteristic of movements of the carpometacarpal joint of thumb?

Ans. The thumb is lotated by 90° on its long axis, relative to other digits. As a result, ventral surface faces medially and dorsal surface laterally. Therefore flexion and extension take place in plane parallel to palm while in other digits, it takes place in planes at right angles to palm.

Q. Why the movements at first carpometacarpal joint are freer than the other corresponding joints?

Ans. Because this has a separate joint cavity.

Q. Why the abduction and adduction are not possible at metacarpophalangeal joint when fingers are flexed?

Ans. (a) Because each metacarpal head is flattened anteriorly and when base of proximal phalanx moves on this flattened surface abduction and adduction become impossible.

(b) The collateral ligament becomes taut in flexion and prevent sideways movement.

Q. What are the attachments of flexor retinaculum?

Ans. *Medial:* Hook of hammate and
Pisiform.

Lateral: Tubercle of trapezium and
Tubercle of scaphoid.

Q. Name the structures passing superficial to the flexor retinaculum.

Ans. (a) Tendon of palmaris longus.
(b) Palmar cutaneous branch of median nerve,
(c) Palmar cutaneous branch of ulnar nerve,
(d) Ulnar nerve and
(e) Ulnar vessels.

Q. Name the structures passing deep to flexor retinaculum.

Ans. (a) Median nerve
(b) Tendons of flexor digitorum sublimis
(c) Tendons of flexor digitorm profundus
(d) Tendon of flexor pollicis longus
(e) Ulnar bursa
(f) Radial bursa

Q. Name the structures piercing flexor retinaculum.

Ans. 1. Flexor carpi radialis and
2. Flexor carpi ulnaris.

Q. Name the structures passing deep to extensor retinaculum.

Ans. The structures deep to extensor retinaculum lie in 6 compartments formed by septa passing from retinaculum to posterior surface of radius.

The structures from lateral to medial side in each compartment are:

I. (a) Abductor pollicis longus and
(b) Extensor pollicis brevis.

II. (a) Extensor carpi radialis longus and
(b) Extensor carpi radialis brevis.

III. Extensor pollicis longus.

IV. (a) Extensor digitorum
(b) Extensor indices
(c) Posterior interosseous nerve and
(d) Anterior interosseous artery.

V. Extensor digiti minimi.

VI. Extensor carpi ulnaris.

Q. What is 'Palmar aponeurosis'?

Ans. It is central part of deep fascia of palm. It improves the grip by fixing the skin of palm. Digital nerves, vessels and tendons pass deep to it, so it protects these.

Q. How fibrous flexor sheaths of fingers are formed? What is their importance?

Ans. These are made up of deep fascia of the fingers, which is thickened and arched to be attached to side of the phalanges and across the base of distal phalanx.

It forms a fascial tunnels which contains long flexor tendons enclosed in digital synovial sheath and it holds the tendons in position during flexion of the digits.

Q. What are the muscles forming the thenar eminence?

Ans. (a) Abductor pollicis brevis

(b) Flexor pollicis brevis

(c) Opponens pollicis

(d) Adductor pollicis.

Q. Name the muscle lying deepest at the thenar eminence?

Ans. Adductor pollicis.

Q. Name the muscles forming the hypothenar eminence?

Ans. (a) Abductor digiti minimi

(b) Flexor digiti minimi

(c) Opponens digiti minimi.

Q. What is Dupuytren's contracture?

Ans. It is thickening and contraction of ulnar side of palmar aponeurosis.

This usually affects ring finger in which proximal and middle phalanx are flexed and cannot be straightened.

Q. What are the differences between lumbricals of hand?

Ans. 4 lumbricals in hand

		Medial two	*Lateral two*
1.	Structure	Bipennate	Unipennate
2.	Nerve supply	Median nerve	Ulnar nerve

Q. Which digit does not have palmar interossei?
Ans. Third digit.

Q. Which digit does not have dorsal interossei?
Ans. First and fifth.

Q. What are the functions of lumbricals and interossei?
Ans. (a) Lumbricals and interossei together bring about
1. Flexion at metacarpophalangeal joint and
2. Extension at interphalangeal joints.

(b) Lumbricals alone are weak flexors of metacarpophalangeal joint.
(c) Palmar interossei are adductors of fingers.
(d) Dorsal interossei are abductors of fingers.

AXILLA

Q. What is the shape of axilla?
Ans. It is a four sided pyramidal shaped space, situated between upper part of arm and chest wall.

Q. What is the direction of apex of axilla?
Ans. It is direct upwards and medially towards the root of neck.

Q. What is 'cervicoaxillay canal'?
Ans. It is a triangular interval bound by:
Arteriorly: Posterior surface of clavicle.
Posteriorly: Superior border of scapula.
Medially: Outer border of first rib.
It corresponds to apex of axilla and through it axillary vessels and brachial plexus enter the axilla from the neck.

Q. What are the contents of the axilla?
Ans. (a) Axillary artery and its branches.
(b) Axillary vein and its tributaries.
(c) Infraclavicular part of the brachial plexus.
(d) Axillary lymph nodes and lymphatics.
(e) Long thoracic and intercostobrachial nerves.
(f) Axillary fat and areolar tissue.

Q. What are the boundaries of axilla?

Ans. (a) *Apex:* Truncated.

(b) *Base:* Skin and axillary fascia.

(c) *Anterior wall:* Pectoralis major, pectoralis minor and clavipectoral fascia.

(d) *Posterior wall:* Subscapularis above, teres major and latissimus dorsi below.

(e) *Medial wall:* Upper four ribs with intercostal muscles, upper part of serratus anterior.

(f) *Lateral wall:* Upper part of shaft of humerus, coracobrachialis, short head of biceps muscle.

ARTERIES OF UPPER LIMB

Q. What is the extent of axillary artery?

Ans. It extends from outer border of first rib to lower border of teres major muscle. It is a continuation of subclavian artery and it continues as brachial artery.

Q. What are the parts of axillary artery?

Ans. Pectoralis minor muscle crosses it and divides it into three parts:

First Part: Proximal to muscle.

Second Part: Posterior to muscle.

Third Part: Distal to muscle.

Q. What are the relations of various nerves with the axillary artery?

Ans. *First part:*

Anterior:

(a) Supraclavicular nerves

(b) Lateral pectoral nerve

(c) Loop of communication between lateral and medial pectoral nerve.

Posterior:

(a) Nerve to serratus arterior

(b) Medial cord of brachial plexus

Lateral: Lateral and posterior cords of brachial plexus.

Second part:

Posterior: Posterior cord of brachial plexus

Medial:

(a) Medial cord of brachial plexus

(b) Medial pectoral nerve

Lateral: Lateral cord of brachial plexus.

Third part:

Anterior: Medial root of median nerve

Posterior: Axillary nerve

Lateral:

(a) Musculocutaneous nerve and lateral root of median nerve in upper part.

(b) Trunk of median nerve in lower part.

Medial:

(a) Medial cutaneous nerve of forearm

(b) Ulnar nerve

(c) Medial cutaneous nerve of arm

Q. What is the relation of various muscles with axillary artery?

Ans. *Anteriorly:*

Pectoralis major to whole artery except lowermost part

Pectoralis minor to second part

Clavipectoral fascia to first part

Posteriorly:

Intercostal muscles of first space and serratus anterior to first part

Subscapularis to second and upper portion of third part. Teres major and tendon of latissimus dorsi to lower portion of third part

Laterally:

Coracobrachialis to second and third part

Q. Which veins cross the axillary artery?

Ans. Cephalic vein and thoracoacromial vein, the tributaries of axillary vein cross the first part.

Q. Name the branches of axillary artery.

Ans. *From first part:* Superior thoracic artery

From second part:

(a) Thoracoacromial artery

(b) Lateral thoracic artery.

From third part:
(a) Subscapular artery
(b) Anterior circumflex humeral artery
(c) Posterior circumflex humeral artery

Q. What is the extent of brachial artery?

Ans. It extends from the lower border of teres major muscle to elbow at the level of neck of radius just medial to tendon of biceps.

Q. What are the nerves related to brachial artery in its course?

Ans.
1. *In upper part of arm:*
   (a) Anteriorly to medial cutaneous nerve of forearm
   (b) Medially, to ulnar nerve
   (c) Laterally, to median nerve.
2. *In middle of arm:* Crossed by median nerve from lateral to medial side.
3. *In lower part of arm:* Medially, median nerve. Posteriorly, it is related to Radial nerve, only in the upper most part.
4. *In elbow:*
   Laterally: Radial nerve
   Medially: Median nerve

Q. Name the branches of brachial artery.

Ans.
1. Muscular branches
2. Profunda brachii artery
3. Superior ulnar collateral
4. Inferior ulnar collateral
5. Nutrient artery to humerus
6. *Terminal branches:* Radial and ulnar.

Q. What is the clinical importance of brachial artery?

Ans. Brachial pulsations are auscultated in front of elbow just medial to tendon of biceps while recording the blood pressure.

Q. Name the branches of profunda brachii artery.

Ans.
(a) Anterior descending
(b) Posterior descending
(c) Ascending branch

Q. Name the branches of radial artery.

Ans. 1. Muscular branches
2. Radial recurrent branch
3. Palmar carpal branch
4. superficial palmar branch
5. Dorsal carpal branch
6. First dorsal metacarpal artery
7. Princeps pollicis artery
8. Radialis indicis artery

Q. Where the pulsations of radial artery are felt?

Ans. At the wrist against the anterior surface of lower end of radius.

Q. Name the branches of ulnar artery.

Ans. (a) Muscular branches
(b) Anterior and posterior ulnar recurrent branches
(c) Palmar and dorsal carpal branches
(d) Common interosseous artery
(e) Superficial and deep palmar branch.

Q. Anterior interosseous artery lies between which muscles?

Ans. Flexor digitorum profundus and flexor pollicis longus.

Q. Name the structure separating the ulnar artery from median nerve at elbow

Ans. Ulnar head of pronator teres.

Q. What are the relations of radial artery in the forearm

Ans. Radial artery lies between flexor carpi radialis and brachioradialis.

Q. What is clinical importance of Allen's test?

Ans. This test is performed to test the patency of the radial or ulnar artery.

Q. Name the arteries forming an anastomosis around the Scapula

Ans. (a) Supracapular artery } Branch of thyrocervical joint
(b) Deep branch of transverse cervical artery } Branch of thyrocervical joint
(c) Circumflex scapular artery, branch of subscapular artery.

Q. How the circulation is carried out when axillary artery is ligated.

Ans. By the collateral channels around the scapula, which connect the first part of subclavian artery with third part of axillary artery.

VENOUS DRAINAGE OF UPPER LIMB

Q. What are the main superficial veins of upper limb?

Ans. (a) *Cephalic (Preaxial) vein:* Begins from lateral end of dorsal venous arch and drains into axillary vein

(b) *Basillic (Post axial) veins:* Begins from medial end of the dorsal venous arch and above the lower border of teres major continues as the axillary vein

(c) *Median cubital vein:* Large communicating vein which shunts blood from cephalic to basilic in 70%.

(d) *Median vein of forearm:* Drains the palmar venous arch and ends in basilic or median cubital veins.

Q. Name the structures lying between axillary artery and vein

Ans. The vein lies anteromedial to the artery. The two are separated by,

(a) Medial cord of brachial plexus
(b) Medial pectoral nerve
(c) Ulnar nerve
(d) Medial cutaneous nerve of forearm

Q. How the venous drainage of upper limb is maintained in axillary vein obstruction?

Ans. By communication between upper part of cephalic vein with the external jugular vein in neck.

Q. What is the clinical importance of median cubital vein?

Ans. It is connected to the deep veins of upper limb through a perforator which pierces the bicipital aponeurosis, which fixes it. So it does not slip away when intravenous injections are given

LYMPHATIC DRAINAGE OF UPPER LIMB

Q. Which is main lymph node of upper limb?

Ans. Lateral group of axillary nodes

Q. What is the area of lymphatic drainage of axillary lymph nodes?

Ans. *Anterior group:* Drains skin and muscles of anterior and lateral walls of trunk upto level of umbilicus and part of breast.

Posterior group: Drains skin and muscles of back of trunk from iliac crest to lower part of neck.

Lateral group: Upper limb

Q. How the axillary lymph nodes drain?

Ans. Anterior, posterior and lateral group drain into central group which in turn drains into apical group. Subclavian lymphatic trunk from apical group drains into thoracic duct on left side and to right lymphatic duct on right side.

BREAST

Q. What is breast?

Ans. It is *modified gland of apocrine type*, which is present in both the sexes, but is rudimentary in males and well developed in females after puberty.

It forms as important accessory organ of female reproductive system.

Q. What is extent of female breast?

Ans. *Superiorly:* 2nd rib

Inferiorly: 6th rib.

Medially: Lateral border of sternum.

Laterally: Mid-axillary line

The superolateral part of gland is prolonged upwards and laterally, pierces the deep fascia at anterior fold of axilla and lies in the axilla at the level of third rib. This process of gland is known as '*Axillary tail of Spence*' and the opening in deep fascia is known as '*Foramen of Langer*'.

Q. What is situation of breast?

Ans. Breast lies in the superficial fascia of pectoral region except for axillary tail which pierces the deep fascia through foramen of Langer and lies in axilla.

Q. What is shape of breast?

Ans. In young adult female, it is hemispherical.
In later life, it is usually pendulous.

Q. What are deep relations of breast?

Ans.
1. Retromammary space of loose areolar tissue. According to former concept of free flow of lymphatics, it was known as *Lake of Marcille.*
2. Pectoral fascia
3. Pectoralis major, serratus anterior and external oblique

Q. What is the structure of breast?

Ans.
1. *Glandular tissue:* This consists of 15-20 lobes. Each lobe consists of several lobules and each lobule consists of a cluster of *alveoli* which open into the smallest branches of lactiferous ducts. These branches unite to form larger branches of duct.
   Each lactiferous duct, drains a lobe of gland and opens at nipple. At the bottom of the nipple each duct is dilated to form a *sinus*. The ducts are arranged radially around the nipple. The glandular tissue is the functional portion of the breast and secretes milk.
2. *Fibrous tissue stroma:* This consists of numerous septa connecting the lobules and supporting them. These septa link the pectoral fascia to the skin of the breast. These are known as '*suspensory ligaments of Cooper*'.
3. *Adipose tissue:* This fills the interalveolar and interductular intervals and accounts for the smooth contour and most of t he bulk of breast.
4. *Skin:*
   (i) *Nipple:* Cylindrical or conical projection directed superolaterally. It lies at the level of 4th intercostal space in nulliparous females

(ii) *Areola:* Pigmented area around nipple. Rose pink in virgins and dark brown or black after pregnancy. The nipple and the subareolar tissue contain smooth muscle but lack the fat.

(iii) *Montgomery's Tubercles:* These are sebaceous glands underlying the areolar skin and are called areolar glands. They enlarge during pregnancy and lactation and form raised tubercles. Oily secretions of these glands lubricates nipple and areola and prevent them from cracking during lactation.

Q. How does the structure of male breast differs from the female breast?

Ans. The male breast is rudimentary. It consist of small ducts without alveoli. There is little supporting fibrous tissue and fat.

Q. What is retromammary space and what is its clinical significance?

Ans. It is a space which lies between the deep aspect of the breast and the fascia covering the pectoralis major. It contains loose areolar tissue and allows the breast some degree of movement on pectoral fascia.

Fixity of the breast to the pectoral fascia and the muscle may occur, by invasion, in advanced carcinoma of breast. This is of great significance in clinical staging of breast carcinoma.

Q. What is the clinical significance of retraction of nipple?

Ans. (a) *Retraction occurring at pregnancy:* It is due to a developmental abnormality. The nipple, for some unknown reason, does not develop with breast.

(b) Recent retraction of nipple may be due to the fibrous contraction of the lactiferous ducts in breast carcinoma or chronic abscess

Q. Why the young breast is protuberant and older breast pendulous?

Ans. The young breast is supported by fibrous tissue strands, *the ligaments of Cooper*, which connect the deep fascia with overlying skin. When these atrophy the organ drops and becomes pendulous.

Q. What is the clinical significance of the dimpling of skin over breast?

Ans. This is due to contraction of ligaments of Cooper. It can occur in chronic infection, after trauma or the breast carcinoma infiltrating the ligaments.

Q. What is arterial supply of breast?

Ans. *Breast is supplied by*:

1. Internal thoracic artery, through its perforating branches in 2nd-6th intercostal space.
2. Lateral thoracic
3. Superior thoracic
4. Acromio-thoracic
5. Lateral branches of posterior intercostal arteries

(2–4: Branches of axillary artery)

Q. What is the venous drainage of breast?

Ans. Veins converge towards the base of nipple where they form an anastomotic venous circle, from where veins run in superficial and deep sets.

(i) Superficial veins drain into internal thoracic and superficial veins of lower neck.
(ii) Deep veins drain into internal thoracic, axillary and posterior intercostal veins.

Q. What is the importance of knowing venous drainage of breast?

Ans.
1. Veins indicate lymphatic pathways because the lymphatics run with the veins
2. Carcinoma of breast can spread through veins
3. As the posterior intercostal veins communicate with the vertebral plexus of veins through which the malignancy can spread to bones and nervous system

Q. What is the nerve supply of breast?

Ans. Breast is supplied by anterior and lateral cutaneous branches of 4th to 6th intercostal nerves. Nerves do not control the secretion of milk. The nerves supplying the glandular tissue are sympathetic.

Q. What is lymphatic drainage of breast?

Ans. (i) *Superficial lymphatics:* Draining the skin over breast except for nipple and arecla. They pass into axillary, internal mammary, supraclavicular and cephalic lymph nodes.

Superficial lymphatics of one side communicate with those of the other side so unilateral malignancy can become bilateral

(ii) *Deep lymphatics:* Drain the parenchyma of breast, nipple and areola.

(a) 75% of lymph drains into axillary lymph nodes mainly anterior group

(b) 20% drains into internal mammary group, which drain the lymph not only from the medial quadrant, but also from lateral quadrant.

(c) 5% drain into posterior intercostal nodes

(d) The *subareolar plexus of Sappy* situated beneath the areola drains the nipple and areola and communicates with the lymphatics of parenchyma

(e) Lymphatics from the deep surface pass through pectoralis major and clavipectoral fascia, to reach apical group of lymph nodes

(f) Lymphatics from the lower and inner quadrants may communicate with subdiaphragmatic and subperiotoneal lymph plexus, after crossing the costal margin and then piercing the anterior abdominal wall through upper part of linea alba. Thus, the carcinoma of breast may spread to the liver and can gravitate through the peritoneal cavity to lie on the pelvic organs, e.g., on ovary, when the condition is known as *Krukenberg's tumour*.

Q. What is the lymphatic drainage of axillary tail?

Ans. It drains into the scapular (anterior) axillary group.

Q. What is Peau d'orange kin?

Ans. Peau d'orange is due to cutaneous lymphatic oedema. Where the infiltrated skin is tethered by the sweat ducts, it cannot swell. The characteristic appearance is like that of orange peel. It is a classical physical sign of advanced carcinoma of breast. It is also seen over an abscess, particularly chronic abscess of the breast.

Q. How the carcinoma breast spreads to the vertebrae?

Ans. By spread through the veins.

Q. What is Cancer en Cuirasse?

Ans. In it, there is persistent, non-pitting oedema of the arm and the affected side of the thoracic wall is studded with carcinomatous nodules and the skin is so infiltrated that it is like the coat of armour. The condition appears in cases where local recurrence after surgery of breast occurs.

Q. How does the breast develop?

Ans. The breast develops as an in vagination of ectoderm of the ventral wall of the body. In the 6th week of inter-uterine life, two longitudinal ectodermal thickening develop, one on each side called *mammary ridge or milk ridge*. This ridge extends from the axilla to the groin, but in the human embryo it persists only in the pectoral region. Ingrowths from the milk ridge gives rise to the glandular tissue, the ducts and alveoli of breasts. The connective tissue supporting the glandular tissue is derived from the surrounding mesenchyme

Q. What is Polymastia (Supernumerary breast)?

Ans. This is congenital anomaly in human in which there are more than one breast on one or both sides. This is due to the persistence of the milk ridge which normally disappears except in the pectoral region.

Q. What is polythelia?

Ans. This is the presence of supernumerary nipples.

Q. What type of incisions is given to drain a breast abscess?

Ans. By a radial incision to avoid cutting across a number of lactiferous ducts

Q. What is the extent of clavipectoral fascia?

Ans. *Vertically:*

Superiorly, splits to enclose subclavius muscle and is attached to the clavicle.

Inferiorly, splits to enclose pectoralis minor and continues as suspensory ligament.

Horizontally:

Medially, attached to first rib, costoclavicular ligament and fascia covering the two intercostal spaces.

Laterally, attached to coacoid process and blends with the coracoclavicular ligament.

Q. Name the structures piercing clavipectoral fascia.

Ans. 1. Lateral pectoral nerve
2. Cephalic vein
3. Thoraco-acromial vessels
4. Lymphatics

BRACHIAL PLEXUS

Q. What is brachial plexus?

Ans. Brachial plexus is formed by the union of the ventral rami of lower four cervical nerves ($C_{5.6.7.8}$) and the greater part of the ventral ramus of the first thoracic nerve (T_1). The fourth cervical nerve usually gives a branch to the fifth cervical and the first thoracic nerve frequently receives one from the second thoracic nerve

Q. What is prefixed and postfixed type of plexus?

Ans. When the branch from C_4 is large, the branch from T_2 is frequently absent and the branch of T_1 is reduced in size. This is prefixed type of plexus. On the other hand, the branch form C_4 may be very small or entirely absent. In the event, the contribution of C_5 is reduced in size but that of T_1 is larger and T_2 is always present. That constitutes postfixed type of plexus

Q. How the banchial plexus forms trunks?

Ans. The C_5 and C_6 join to form upper trunk, C_7 forms the middle trunk and C_8 and T_1 join to form the lower trunk.

Each trunk divides into ventral and dorsal division, which ultimately supply anterior and posterior aspect of upper limb

Q. How the cords of brachial plexus are formed?

Ans. Lateral cord is formed by union of ventral division of the upper and middle trunks. The medial cord is formed by the ventral divisions of lower trunk. Posterior cord is formed by union of dorsal divisions of all the three trunks.

Q. What are the branches of roots of brachial plexus?

Ans. (a) Long thoracic nerve (Nerve to serratus anterior) $C_{5,6,7}$.

(b) Dorsal scapular nerve (Nerve to rhomboids) C_5.

Q. What are the branches of trunks of brachial plexus?

Ans. (a) Supracapular nerve ($C_{5,6}$).

(b) Nerve to subclavius ($C_{5,6}$)

Q. What are the branches of lateral cord of brachial plexus?

Ans.
1. Lateral pectoral nerve
2. Lateral root of median nerve
3. Musculocutaneous nerve

Q. What is the main nerve supply of pectoralis major?

Ans. Lateral pectoral nerve

Q. What are the branches of medial cord of brachial plexus?

Ans.
a. Medial root of median nerve
b. Medial pectoral nerve
c. Ulnar nerve
d. Medial cutaneous nerve of arm
e. Medial cutaneous nerve of forearm.

Q. What are the branches of posterior cord of brachial plexus?

Ans.
a. Radial nerve
b. Axillary nerve
c. Thoracodorsal nerve (Nerve to latissimus dorsi)
d. Upper subscapsular nerve
e. Lower subscapsular nerve

Q. What is main nerve supply of pectoralis minor?

Ans. Medial pectoral nerve

Q. What is the distribution of suprascapular nerve?

Ans. *Muscular:* Supraspinatus
Infraspinatus
Articular: Shoulder joint
Acromioclavicular joint

Q. What is Erb's point?

Ans. It is the junction of the ventral primary rami of C_5 and C_6 forming the upper trunk of the brachial plexus. The trunk being short, the suprascapular nerve and nerve to subclavius which arise directly from it and the anterior and posterior divisions of trunk all lie close to the Erb's point and may be involved in any injury at this point.

Q. What is Erb's paralysis?

Ans. It is the paralysis resulting from a lesion of the upper trunk at the Erb's point. It is caused by the forcible downward traction of the shoulder with lateral displacement of the head to the other side.

In this lesion, the area of distribution of C_5 and C_6 is affected and most commonly the muscles supplied by C_5 are involved. The deltoid, biceps, brachialis, brachioradialis and sometimes supraspinatus, infraspinatus and supinator are paralysed. The affected limb assumes a characteristic '*waiter's tip*' *position*.

(a) The arm hangs simply by the side due to paralysis of the deltoid and supraspinatus and is rotated medially, due to paralysis of infraspinatus
(b) The elbow is extended due to paralysis of the biceps and brachialis and imposed action of the extensors of elbow.
(c) The forearm is pronated due to paralysis of the biceps and supinator
(d) The wrist is slightly flexed due to weak wrist extensors.

Q. What is Klumpke's paralysis?

Ans. This is a paralysis resulting from the lesion of the lower trunk (C_8 and T_1 nerve roots). It is caused by forceful upward traction of the arm. The area of distribution mainly of T_1 is involved, i.e., all the intrinsic muscles of the hand are affected and flexors of wrist are affected due to C_8 root involvement.

(a) The hand assumes a characteristic deformity described as *claw hand*. In this, the metacarpo-phalangeal joints are hyperextended due to unopposed action of the long extensors as the lumbricals and interossei are paralysed while the inter-phalangeal joints are flexed due to unopposed actions of the long flexors of the fingers.

(b) There is sensory loss along the ulnar side of the hand, forearm and arm

(c) There may also be Horner's syndrome characterised by moisis, ptosis, anhydrosis and anophthalmos

Q. What is the clinical importance of postfixed type of brachial plexus?

Ans. The T_2 root has to curve up over the first rib to form the brachial plexus. This results in greater pressure on T_2 nerve root in post fixed brachial plexus as compared to normal. Hence symptoms associated cervical rib can be present in absence of such a rib.

Q. What is the cause of the referred pain to the skin over shoulder?

Ans. This is due to inflammation of the diaphragmatic pelura or peritoneum, (usually occurring in cholecystitis and splenic infarction) which has the same segmental nerve supply (C_4) via phrenic nerve as the shoulder skin via the lateral supraclavicular nerve.

Q. What is 'Crutch paralysis'?

Ans. It is due to the damage to the brachial plexus in the axilla from the pressure of crutch. In these, the radial nerve is frequently implicated and ulnar nerve suffers next in frequency.

Q. What is 'Saturday night palsy'?

Ans. This is radial nerve palsy due to the prolonged pressure on the nerve in the spiral groove of the humerus. This occurs when a drunkard falls into sleep (on Saturday night!) with his arm hanging over the back of chair.

In the morning, he is suffering from the wrist drop which is temporary.

Q. What is 'Winging of scapula'?

Ans. This is clinical condition in which the inferior angle and the medial border of the scapula becomes unduly prominent. It occurs in the paralysis of long thoracic nerve (Nerve of Bell) which supplies serratus anterior. It can be demonstrated by asking the patient to push against the wall with outstretched hands. The scapula on affected side becomes winged due to unopposed action of the rhomboids and levator scapulae, while the paralysed serratus anterior is not contracting.

Q. Name the clinical conditions in which the axillary nerve is likely to be injured.

Ans. (i) Fracture of surgical neck of humerus
(ii) Dislocation of shoulder joint.

Q. What will be the effects of complete damage of the axillary nerve?

Ans.
1. There is paralysis of the deltoid and teres minor. Paralysis of deltoid causes inability to abduct the shoulder joint while the wasting of the muscles causes undue prominence of the acromion. Paralysis of teres minor is not easily demonstrated clinically.
2. There will be sensory loss over the lower part of deltoid.

RADIAL NERVE

Q. What is origin of radial nerve?

Ans. It is a branch of posterior cord of brachial plexus with a root value of $C_{5.6.7.8}\ T_1$.

Q. What are the branches and distribution of radial nerve?

Ans. (a) *Muscular branches*: To
1. Triceps
2. Anconeus

3. Brachialis, only lateral part
4. Brachioradialis and
5. Extensor carpi radialis longus

(b) *Cutaneous branches:*

1. Lower lateral cutaneous nerve of arm
2. Posterior cutaneous nerve of forearm
3. Posterior cutaneous nerve of arm
4. Dorsal digital branches from superficial terminal branch

(c) *Articular branches:* To elbow and wrist joint.

Q. What are the structures supplied by posterior interosseous nerve?

Ans. Muscular branches:

(a) Extensor carpi radialis brevis
(b) Supinator
(c) Extensor digitorum
(d) Extensor digiti minimi
(e) Extensor carpi ulnaris
(f) Extensor pollicis longus
(g) Extensor indicis
(h) Abductor pollicis longus
(i) Extensor pollicis brevis

Q. What is the commonest site of radial nerve injury? What are the common causes of lesion?

Ans. In the region of radial (spiral) groove of humerus. The common causes of injury are:

(a) Fracture of shaft of humerus
(b) Intramuscular injections in arm

Q. What are the effects of the lesion of radial nerve in the spiral groove?

Ans. (i) Triceps is not paralysed since the branches supplying arise from the radial nerve more proximally.

(ii) There is *wrist drop, i.e.*, hand is flexed at wrist and it lies flaccid due to the paralysis of the extensors of the wrist. The fingers are also flexed and when an attempt is made to extend them, the last two phalanges only will be extended, through the action of lumbricals and interrossei.

(iii) Supination is completely lost when the forearm is extended on the arm, but is possible to a certain extent if the forearm is flexed to allow effective action of the biceps.

Q. What will be the effect of cutting the radial nerve just below the elbow?

Ans. *Sensory loss:* It is marked on the lateral part of the dorsum of the hand.

Motor loss:

(i) Wrist drop
(ii) Loss of power of supination
(iii) Extension of elbow is retained because of the intact triceps
(iv) Flexion of elbow in normal position will also be retained because of intact biceps brachii and brachioradialis.

Q. What is the 'high' and 'low' radial nerve palsy?

Ans. When radial nerve is damaged above the origin of nerve to brachioradialis which arises above the elbow joint then it is called 'high' radial nerve palsy.

When radial nerve is damaged below the origin of nerve to brachioradialis then it is called 'low' radial nerve palsy. The brachioradialis is not paralysed and cause flexion of the elbow joint in the mid prone position which when elbow is flexed against resistance becomes prominent, can be felt superficially on lateral aspect of the forearm.

MUSCULOCUTANEOUS NERVE

Q. What is the origin of musculocutaneous nerve?

Ans. It is a branch of lateral cord of brachial plexus, arising at the lower border of pectoralis minor ($C_{5,6,7}$).

Q. What are the branches of musculocutaneous nerve?

Ans. *Muscular:* To,

(a) Coracobrachilais
(b) Biceps and
(c) Brachialis

Cutaneous: It continues as lateral cutaneous nerve of forearm and supplies skin of lateral side of forearm.
Articular: To elbow joint
Communicating: To radial nerve, posterior cutaneous nerve of forearm and palmar cutaneous branch of median nerve.

Q. What will be the affect of lesion of the musculocutaneous nerve.

Ans. *Motor loss:* There will be paralysis of the biceps, coracobrachial is and the medial part of brachialis, the lateral part being supplied by the radial nerve.

Effects:

(i) Flexion of the elbow joint will be weak but is still possible,
  (a) with the forearm supinated due to the action of the unaffected lateral part of brachialis and superficial flexors and
  (b) in the prone or midprone position by the brachioradialis and extensor carpi radialis longus.

(ii) There will be very weak supination with the elbow flexed at 90°.

(iii) There will be loss of biceps jerk

(iv) There will be muscles atrophy.

Sensory loss: Will be present over the lateral half of the forearm but the area will be less due to overlapping of the intact adjacent cutaneous nerves.

MEDIAN NERVE

Q. What is the origin of median nerve?

Ans. Median nerve is formed by the union of a medial root (C_8, T_1) from medial cord and lateral root ($C_{5,6,7}$) from lateral cord.

Q. Name the branches and structures supplied by median nerve?

Ans. *In arm:*

(a) Muscular branch to pronator teres
(b) Vascular branches to brachial artery

In forearm:

(a) Muscular branches to flexor carpi radials, palmaris longus, flexor digitorum superficialis.

(b) *Anterior interosseous branch* to flexor pollicis longus, lateral half of flexor digitorum profundus, pronator quadratus and to distal radio-ulnar and wrist joints.

(c) Palmar cutaneous branch, to skin over thenar eminence and middle of the palm.

(d) Articular branch to elbow and proximal radio-ulnar joints

(e) Vascular branches to radial and ulnar arteries.

(f) Communicating branch to ulnar nerve

In hand:

(a) Muscular branches to abductor pollicis brevis, flexor policis brevis, opponens pollicis and first and second lumbrical

(b) Cutaneous branches to skin of lateral 3½ digits (Palmar digital branches).

Q. What will be the effect of a lesion of the median nerve at the wrist?

Ans. 1. *Motor loss:* There will be paralysis of the thenar muscles and the 1st and 2nd lumbricals.

Effect:

(i) There will be loss of opposition of the thumb due to paralysis of the opponens pollicis

(ii) Abduction of the thumb will not be greatly affected due to intact abductor pollicis longus which is supplied by the radial nerve

(iii) Paralysis and wasting of the thenar muscles and unopposed extension by extensor pollicis longus and adduction by adductor pollicis will be rise to *'ape-thumb' deformity*.

2. *Sensory loss:* There will be loss of sensation over the thumb, adjacent 3½ fingers and the radial two thirds of the palm.

Effect: The sensory loss will prevent the accurate and delicate adjustments which the hand makes in response to tactile stimuli.

Q. What is 'Carpal tunnel' syndrome?

Ans. This is a neuropathy resulting from compression of median nerve as it passes beneath the flexor retinaculum through carpal tunnel.

It causes:

(a) *Motor loss:* Progressive weakness and wasting of thenar muscle

(b) *Sensory loss:* In lateral 3½ digits.

ULNAR NERVE

Q. What is the origin of ulnar nerve?

Ans. It arises from medial cord of brachial plexus C_8, T_1.

Q. What are the branches of ulnar nerve?

Ans. *In forearm:*

Muscular: To flexor carpi ulnaris and medial half of flexor digitorum profundus.

Palmar and dorsal cutaneous branches.

In hand:

Muscular:

(a) *By deep terminal branch:* Abductor digiti minimi, flexor digiti minimi, opponens digiti minimi, medial two lumbricals, palmar and dorsal interossei and adductor pollicis

(b) Palmaris brevis by palmar cutaneous or *superficial terminal branch.*

Articular: To elbow joint.

Skin: Medial 1½ fingers by palmar digital branches.

Q. What will be the effect of a lesion of the ulnar nerve at the wrist?

Ans. 1. *Motor loss:* There will be paralysis of all the intrinsic muscles of the hand (except those supplied by the median nerve), i.e., all interossei, 3rd and 4th lumbricals, hypothenar muscles and adductor pollicis.

Effect:

(i) There will be '*Mani-en-griff*' deformity or '*clawing*' of the ring and little fingers. These fingers are hyperextended at the metacarpo-phalangeal joints (due to the unopposed action of the extensor digitorum as the 3rd and 4th lumbricals and all the interossei are paralysed) and flexed at the interphalangeal joints (due to the unopposed action of the long flexors).

(ii) Abduction of 2nd to 5th fingers will be weak due to paralysis of the dorsal interossei and abductor digiti minimi.

(iii) There will be loss of power of adduction of the fingers due to paralysis of the palmar interossei.

(iv) There will be loss of power of adduction of the thumb due to paralysis of the adductor pollicis.

(v) There will be wasting of the hypothenar eminence in long standing injuries

(vi) There will be hollowing between the metacarpal bones, clearly apparent on the dorsum, due to atrophy of the interossei muscles in long standing injuries.

2. *Sensory loss:*

(i) There will be sensory loss on the medial side of the palm and the palmar surfaces of the little and the medial half of the ring fingers and on the dorsal aspect of the distal and middle phalanges of these fingers

(ii) There will be no sensory loss over the dorsum of the hand as the dorsal cutaneous branch of the ulnar nerve will escape the injury. If the nerve is damaged proximal to the origin of this branch, then there will also be sensory loss over the dorsum of the hand.

Q. What will be the effect of a lesion of the ulnar nerve at the elbow?

Ans. 1. *Motor loss:*

(i) Same as when the nerve is damaged at the wrist.

(ii) There will also be paralysis of the medial half of the flexor digitorum profundus supplying the little and ring fingers and of the flexor carpi ulnaris.

Effect:

(i) Same as when the nerve is damaged the wrist. 'Clawing' of the ring and little fingers will be less marked as their distal phalanges are not flexed due to paralysis of only the medial half of the fixor digitorum profundus.

(ii) Loss of power in the flexor carpi ulnaris will result in weak flexion with radial deviation of the wrist.

2. Sensory loss will be present over the ulnar 1½ fingers and the hand.
3. Vasomotor and trophic changes will be present in the skin over the hypothenar eminence and little finger which will appear cold and dry and at times discoloured. The nail of the little finger may be deformed.

SCAPULAR SPACES

Q. What are the boundaries and contents of Quadrangular space?

Ans. *Boundaries:*

Superior:

(a) Subscapularis
(b) Capsule of shoulder joint
(c) Teres minor

Inferior: Teres major
Medial: Long head of triceps
Lateral: Surgical neck of humerus

Contents:

(a) Axillary nerve
(b) Posterior circumflex humeral vessels.

Q. What are the boundaries and contents of upper and lower triangular space?

Ans. *Upper triangular space:*

Boundaries:

Superior: Teres minor
Subscapularis
Lateral: Long head of triceps
Inferior: Teres major.

Contents: Circumflex scapular artery

Lower triangular space:

Boundaries:

Superior: Teres major

Medial: Long head of triceps
Lateral: Medial border of humerus

Contents:

i. Profunda brachii vessels
ii. Radial nerve

Q. What are the boundaries of `Triangle of auscultation?

Ans. *Medial:* Lateral border of trapezius
Lateral: Medial border of scapula
Below: Upper border of latissimus dorsi
Floor:

i. 7th rib and 6th and 7th intercostal spaces.
ii. Rhomboideus major and latissimus dorsi

Q. What is the clinical importace of `Triangle of auscultation?

Ans. It is the only part of the back which is not covered with muscles and breath sounds are better heard there

SPACES OF THE HAND

Q. Name the spaces of hand.

Ans. (a) *Palmar spaces:*

1. Superficial pulp spaces of the fingers
2. Synovial tendon sheats of 2nd, 3rd and 4th fingers
3. Ulnar bursa
4. Radial bursa
5. Midpalmar space
6. Thenar space.

(b) Dorsal spaces:

1. Dorsal subaponeurotic space
2. Dorsal subcutaneous space.

(c) Forearm space of Parona

Q. What are the characteristic features of the pulp space of fingers?

Ans.
1. Front of distal phalanx is covered with subcutaneous fat.
2. Dense fibrous processes bind the skin to the periosteum and divide fat into compartments.

Q. Why the infections of pulp space of fingers are painful?

Ans. Because it cannot expand due to fibrous processes attaching skin to periosteum and thus little swelling causes much increase in tension.

Q. Why the infections of pulp space of fingers cause necrosis of distal 4/5 of terminal phalanx?

Ans. Because of distal 4/5 receives its blood supply fron arteries which traverse fibrous processes and increase in tension due to infection causes their occlusion and proximal 1/5 escapes necrosis because it receives its blood supply by vessels which do not traverse fibrous processes.

Q. Why the infections of little finger and thumb are more dangerous?

Ans. Because the synovial sheath of little finger is continuous with ulnar bursa and that of thumb with radial bursa so, the infections of these can spread of the forearm space of parona.

Q. What is the position of dorsal spaces?

Ans. The subcutaneous space lies deep to skin and subaponeurotic space depp to extensor tendons on dorsal aspect of hand.

Q. What is forearm space of Parona' and its clinical importance?

Ans. It is space between long flexor tendons and pronator quadratus. Proximally, upward extent is limited by origin of flexor digitorum superficialis and inferiorly, it extends upto upper border of flexor retinaculum. The proximal parts of flexor tendons synovial sheath protrude into it.

Clinical importance: It may be infected by the extension of synovial sheath infections from ulnar or radial bursa, leading to hour glass swelling.

Q. What is position and clinical importance of mid-palmar and thenar space?

Ans. These are potential spaces deep to palmar aponeurosis and flexor tendons.

Midpalmar space: Situated under inner half of hollow of palm

Thenar space: Situated under outer half of hollow of palm

Clinical importance: They become infected in wounds of palm and synovial sheath infections. They frequently communicate with each other, so infection can pass from one to the other.

Q. Why the collection of fluid is more on dorsal surface of hand in infections of palmar aspect of fingers?

Ans. Skin on dorsum of fingers and hand is loose, therefore fluid readily collects beneath it. But on the palm of hand, there is little subcutaneous tissue and skin is adherent to underlying palmar fascia.

Lower Limb

BONES OF LOWER LIMB

HIP BONE

Q. What are the different parts of a hip bone?

Ans. The hip bone is made up of three parts, the *ilium* superiorily, *ischium* postereo-inferiorly and *pubis* antero-inferiorly. The three parts join to form a cup shaped hollow articular surface, the *acetabulum.*

Q. How will you determine to which side the hip bone belongs?

Ans. In a hip bone, the acetabulum is directed laterally and the flat ilium forms upper part of bone, lying above the acetabulum. the obturator foramen lies below the acetabulum.

Q. What is the normal anatomical position of the hip bone in the body?

Ans. (a) Pubic tubercle and anterior superior iliae spine lie in the same vertical plane.

(b) The pelvic surface of the body of pubis is directed backwards and upwards.

(c) The ischial spine and upper border of symphysis pubis lie in same horizontal plane and

(d) Symphysis pubis lies in the median plane.

Q. What is the level through which the highest point of the iliac crest passes (intercrestal plane)?

Ans. The intercrestal plane passes at the level of interval between the spines of L_3 and L_4 vertebrae.

Q. What is the clinical importance of intercrestal plane?

Ans. In clinical practice, lumbar puncture is done between the L_3 and L_4 vertebrae.

Q. What are the structures attached to the anterior superior iliac spine?

Ans. It provides:

(a) attachment to the lateral end of inguinal ligament and

(b) origin of sartorius.

Q. Name the structures attached to the iliac crest.

Ans. Anterior 2/3 of iliac crest has:

(i) *Outer lip* which provides

(a) Attachment of fascia lata,

(b) Origin of tensor fasciae lata,

(c) Insertion to external oblique muscle and

(d) Origin to lattisimus dorsi just behind the highest point.

(ii) *Intermediate area* provides origin to internal oblique muscle.

(iii) *Inner lip* provides

(a) Origin to transversus abdominis,

(b) Attachment to fascia iliaca and fascia transversalis,

(c) Origin to quadratus lumoborum in posterior 1/3 and

(d) Attachment to thoracolumbar fascia.

Posterior 1/3 segment of iliac crest has:

(i) *Lateral slope:* Origin of gluteus maximus.

(ii) *Medial slope:* Origin of erector spinae.

(iii) *Medial margin:* Interosseous and dorsal sacroiliac ligaments.

Q. Name the structures attached to anterior inferior iliac spine.

Ans. Anterior inferior iliac spine gives:

(a) Origin to straight head of rectus femoris in superior half and

(b) Attachment to iliofemoral ligament in inferior half.

Q. Name the structures attached to posterior borde of ilium.

Ans. It provides:

(a) Attachment to upper fibres of sacrotuberous ligament and

(b) Origin to fibres of piriformis.

Q. What are the structures attached to gluteal surface of ilium?

Ans. (a) Gluteus medius arises between anterior and posterior gluteal lines.

(b) Gluteus minimus arises between anterior and inferior gluteal line.

(c) Gluteus maximus (upper fibres) arise behind the posterior gluteal line.

(d) Below inferior gluteal line reflected head of rectus femoris arises.

Q. Name the structures attached to the pubic tubercle.

Ans. (i) Medial end of inguinal ligament.

(ii) Ascending loops of cremaster muscle.

Q. Name the structures attached to the crest of pubis.

Ans. (i) Lateral head of rectus abdominis (origin)

(ii) Pyramidalis (origin).

Medial head of rectus abdominis arises from anterior pubic ligament.

Q. What are the structures attached to pectineal line?

Ans. The structures attached to pectineal line are:

1. Conjoint tendon and lacunar ligament at medial end.
2. Pectineal ligament lateral to lacunar ligament.
3. Origin of pectineus muscle and fascia covering it, fron the whole length.
4. Insertion of psoas minor.

Q. Name the structures attached to ischial spine.

Ans. The structures attached to ischial spine are:

(a) Sacrospinous ligament

(b) Origin of coccygeus and levator ani.

(c) Origin of superior gemellus

Q. What are the structures attached to ischial tuberosity?

Ans. From upper area of ischial tuberosity arise semimembranous superolaterally and semitendinosus and long head of biceps femoris superomedially.

From lower lateral area abductor magnus arise.

Q. What are the nerves related to hip bone?

Ans. (a) Sciatic nerve related to lower margin of greater sciatic notch.

(b) Obturator nerve in the obturator canal.
(c) Nerve to obturator internus crosses the base of ischial spine.
(d) Pudendal nerve crosses base of ischial spine.
(e) Nerve to quadratus femoris runs on ischium as it crosses the greater sciatic notch.

FEMUR

Q. What is the normal anatomical position of the femur in the body?

Ans. The head of femur is directed medially, upwards and slightly forwards and the shaft is obliquely downwards and medially, so that the two condyles at lower surface lie in same ~~the horizontal~~ plane.

Q. What is the arterial supply of the head of femur?

Ans. The medial part near fovea, supplied by medial epiphyseal arteries derived from ascending branch of medial circumflex femoral artery and posterior division of obturator artery.

The lateral part of head is supplied by lateral epiphyseal arteries derived from lateral circumflex femoral artery.

Q. What is the nutrient artery of the femur?

Ans. It is derived from second perforating artery.

Q. What is angle of anterversion?

Ans. The angle of anteversion (angle of femoral torsion) is the angle between the transverse axes of upper and lower ends of femur. It is about 15 degrees.

Q. Name the structures attached to intertrochanteric line of femur.

Ans. The following structures are attached to intertrochanteric line:
(a) Capsular ligament of hip joint
(b) Iliøfemoral ligament
(c) Upper fibres of vastus lateralis and vastus medialis.

Q. Which muscle is inserted into trochanteric fossa?
Ans. Obturator externus.

Q. Which muscle is inserted in gluteal tuberosity?
Ans. Deep fibres of gluteus maximus.

Q. What is the origin of popliteus muscle?
Ans. From anterior part of groove on lateral aspect of lateral condyle of femur.

Q. What is the importance of ossification centre for lower end of femur?
Ans. The ossification centre for lower end of femur appears at end of 9th month of intrauterine life (the day of birth). It is of medicolegal importance in cases of newly born child found dead to decide whether it was viable or not.

Q. What is characteristic of primary ossification centre of femur?
Ans. It is the second long bone in body to start ossifying.

Q. Why the fractures of neck of femur, leads to the necrosis of the head?
Ans. Because it will interrupt the blood supply to the head which is derived from:
(a) Vessels travelling up from diaphysis
(b) Vessels in the retinacula of the hip capsule.

Q. Why the intracapsular fracture of the neck of the femur are more dangerous than extracapsular fracture?
Ans. The intracapsular fracture interrupts the blood supply, to the femoral head resulting in necrosis whereas in the extracapsular fracture, the blood supply to the head remains unaffected and so there is no danger of avascular necrosis.

Q. What is Coxa vara?
Ans. In this condition the angle between the femoral neck and shaft is decreased i.e., less than 160°. This results from adduction fractures.

Q. What is Coxa valga?
Ans. Increase in the angle between femoral neck and shaft due to abduction fractures.

Q. At which level fracture of shaft of femur is dangerous?

Ans. Fracture of the lower end of femur are dangerous because proximal edge of the distal fragment is tilted backwards by the gastroenemius, which tears the popliteal artery which lies directly behind it.

TIBIA AND FIBULA

Q. Name the structures attached to the intercondylar area of tibia.

Ans. From before backwards, it provides attachment to:

(a) Anterior horn of medial meniscus,
(b) Anterior cruciate ligament,
(c) Anterior horn of lateral meniscus,
(d) Posterior horn of lateral meniscus
(e) Posterior horn of medial meniscus
(f) Posterior cruciate ligament.

Q. What are the structures related to anterior surface of lower end of tibia?

Ans. From medial to lateral side it is related to tibialis anterior, extensor hallucis longus, anterior tibial vessels, deep peroneal nerve and extensor digitorum longus.

Q. What are the structures related to the posterior surface of lower end of tibia?

Ans. From medial to lateral side it is realted to tibialis posterior, flexor digitorum longus, posterior tibial artery, tibial nerve and flexor hallucis longus.

Q. What is the arterial supply of tibia?

Ans. Nutrient artery to tibia is a branch of the posterior tibial artery. It is the largest nutrient artery in the body.

Q. Although the tibia is one of the commonest sites of acute osteomyelitis but knee joint is not involved. Explain?

Ans. The knee joint is not involved because the capsule is attached near articular margins of tibia, proximal to epiphyseal line.

Q. The fracture of tibia is slow healing. Why?

Ans. The tibia is commonly fractured at the junction of upper 2/3 and lower 1/3 of its shaft, where it is most slender and this site is poorly supplied by blood vessels.

Q. How will you determine the side to which the fibula belongs?

Ans. The head is slightly expanded in all directions and lateral malleolus is expanded anteroposteriorly and is flattened from side to side. The medial side of lower end bears a triangular articular facet anteriorly and malleolar fossa posteriorly.

Q. Which structure lies between two heads of origin of peroneus longus?

Ans. Common peroneal nerve.

Q. Name the structures attached to malleolar fossa.

Ans. Malleolar fossa provides attachment to posterior talofibular and posterior tibiofibular ligament.

Q. Fibula violates the general rule of ossification. Explain.

Ans. Normally in a long bone, growing end of a long bone ossifies first and unites with the shaft last while the non-growing end ossifies last and fuses with the shaft first. But in fibula, the ossification centre for non-growing end, i.e., lower end appears first but does not fuse last. This occurs because:

(i) the upper epiphysis (fuses last) is the growing end of the bone and

(ii) centre for lower end appears first because it is a pressure epiphysis.

Q. What are the function of fibula?

Ans. (a) It provides origin to muscles.

(b) It acts as a pulley for the tendons of peroneus longus and brevis.

(c) It forms a part of the ankle joint.

(d) It helps to increase the stability of ankle joint by lateral malleolus and ligaments attached to it.

PATELLA

Q. What is the function of patella?

Ans. The patella improves the leverage of the quadriceps femoris by increasing the angulation of the line of pull on the leg.

Q. How the stability of the patella is increased?

Ans. Due to outward angulation between long axes of thign and leg the patella has a tendency to dislocate outwards. This is prevented by:

(i) *Muscular factor:* Insertion of vastus medialis on medial border of patella extends of a lower level than that of the vastus lateralis laterally.

(ii) *Bony factor:* Lateral edge of patellar articular surface of femur is deeper than medial edge.

Q. What are the different sesamoid bones present in the lower limb?

Ans. The following sesamoid bones are present in the lower limb:

(a) Patella, articulates with femur.

(b) Two small sesamoid bones in the tendons of flexor hallucis brevis, articulate with the head of the first metatarsal bone.

(c) One in the peroneus longus tendon, articulates with cuboid.

(d) Others may be present in the tendons of tibialis anterior, lateral head of gastrocnemius and gluteus maximus.

Q. What is 'Febella'?

Ans. It is a small, rounded seasamoid bone present in the lateral head of gastrocnemics. It articulates with the posterior surface of the lateral condyle of femur.

BONES OF FOOT

Q. Name the tarsal bone of foot.

Ans. (a) *Proximal row:* Talus, calcaneum,

(b) *Distal row:* Cuboid and medial, intermediate and lateral cuneiform.

Navicular is interposed between the two rows

Q. Name the structures attached to medial tubercle of calcaneum.

Ans. *Medially:*

(a) Origin of abductor hallucis

(b) Flexor retinaculum.

Anteriorly:

(a) Origin of flexor digitorum brevis

(b) Plantar aponeurosis

Q. Name the structures attached to lateral tubercle of calcaneum.

Ans. Origin of abductor digiti minimi.

Q. Name the tendons related to peroneal trochlea of calcaneum.

Ans. *Above:* Tendon of peroneus brevis

Below: Tendon of peroneus longus.

Q. What are the structures attached to sustentaculum tali?

Ans. To its medial margin are attached

(a) Spring ligament, anteriorly

(b) Slip from tibialis posterior, in middle

(c) Superficial fibres of deltoid ligament, along its whole length and

(d) Medial talocalcanean ligament, posteriorly.

Q. What is the structure attached to tuberosity of navicular bone?

Ans. (a) Insertion for tibialis posterior.

Q. Name the structures related to plantar groove of cuboid.

Ans. (a) Through groove pass tendon of peroneus longus.

(b) To posterior ridge, deep fibres of long plantar ligament.

Q. At what time the ossification centre for cuboid appears?

Ans. Just before or after birth.

Q. What are the differences between metacarpal and metatarsal?

Ans.

Metacarpal	Metatarsal
(a) *Head and shaft:* Prismoid	Flattened from side to side
(b) *Shaft:* Uniform thickness	Tapers distally
(c) *Dorsal surface of shaft:* Elongated, flat triangular area	Uniformly convex
(d) *Base:* Irregular	Cuts sharply and obliquely

Q. What are the "Accessory bones"?

Ans. These are separate small pieces of bone which have not fused with the main bone e.g.,

(a) Os trigonum (posterior tubercle of talus) and

(b) Os Vesalianum (tuberosity of fifth metatarsal).

Q. What is 'bunion'?

Ans. It is inflammed adventitial bursa over the head of first metatarsal bone.

JOINTS OF LOWER LIMB

HIP JOINT

Q. What is the type of hip joint?

Ans. Hip joint is a ball and socket type of synovial joint.

Q. What are the factors which increase the stability of the hip joint?

Ans. The stability of hip joint is increased by the following factors:

(a) Depth of acetabulum with a narrow mouth, made by acetabular labrum.

(b) Tension and strength of ligaments.

(c) Strength of the surrounding muscles.

(d) Length and obliquity of neck of femur.

The wide range of mobility depends upon the neck of femur which is narrower than the equatorial diameter of the head.

Q. What is the attachment of ligament of the head of femur?

Ans. It is attached laterally to fovea on head of femur and medially to two ends of acetabular notch and to transverse ligament.

Q. What are the ligaments strengthening the capsule of hip joint?

Ans. (a) Iliofemoral ligament: Strongest, Y-shaped ligament.
(b) Pubofemoral ligament
(c) Ischiofemoral ligament.

Q. What are the relations of the hip joint?

Ans. The relations of the hip joint are:
(a) *Anteriorly:* Lateral fibres are pectineus, iliopsoas, straight head of rectus femoris.
(b) *Posteriorly:* Quadratus femoris covering obturator externus and ascending branch of medial circumflex femoral artery, the piriformis, obturator internus with two gemelli separate the sciatic nerve from the nerve to quadratus femoris.
(c) *Superior:* Reflected head of rectus femoris covered by gluteus minimus.
(d) *Inferior:* Lateral fibres of pectineus and obturator externus.

Q. What is the axis of different movements of hip joint?

Ans. (a) For rotation, vertical axis passing through the centre of head of femur and its lateral condyle.
(b) Extension and flexion, occur around a transverse axis.
(c) Adduction and abduction, occur around an anteroposterior axis.

Q. What is the range of movements at the hip joint?

Ans. Flexion is limited by contact of thigh with anterior abdominal wall.
Adduction is limited by contact with opposite limb.
Range of other movements: Lateral rotation 60°, Medial rotation 25°, Abduction 50° and extension 15°.

Q. What are the nerves supplying the hip joint?

Ans. The hip joint is supplied by:

(i) Femoral nerve, through nerve to rectus femoris,
(ii) Anterior division of obturator nerve,
(iii) Accessory obturator nerve,
(iv) Nerve to quadratus femoris and
(v) Superior gluteal nerve.

Q. What are the different muscles producing extension of the hip joint?

Ans. Gluteus maximus and hamstrings.

Q. Which muscles produce abduction of the hip joint?

Ans. *Chief muscles:* Gluteus medius and minimus.
Accessory muscles: Tensor fasciae latae and sartorius.

Q. What is Trendelenburg test?

Ans. This test is employed for testing the stability of the hip joint. A positive test indicates a defect in osseo-muscular stability especially abductors of hip joint and the patient has a "lurching" gait. If the patient is asked to stand on one leg. If the abductors of thigh are paralysed on that side, they will be unable to sustain the pelvis against the body weight and pelvis tilts downwards on unsupported side.

Q. Name the adductors of hip joint.

Ans.
1. Adductor longus
2. Adductor brevis
3. Adductor magnus
4. Gracilis
5. Pectineus.

Q. Name the medial rotators of hip joint.

Ans. (a) Gluteus medius and minimus
(b) Tensor fasciae latae
(c) Adductor longus, brevis and magnus.

Q. Name the flexors of hip joint.

Ans. *Mainly:* Psoas major, iliacus, rectus femoris
Accessory muscles: Adductors are also flexors of hip joint.

Q. What is the cause of Weaver's bottom?

Ans. Inflammation of bursa over ischial tuberosity.

Q. In which injury of the hip joint sciatic nerve is likely to be damaged?

Ans. It is likely to be injured in the posterior dislocation of the hip joint associated with fracture of the posterior lip of the acetabulum, to which the nerve is closely related.

KNEE JOINT

Q. What type of joint is the knee joint?

Ans. Compound synovial joint, having

(a) *Condylar synovial joint:* Between the condyles of femur and tibia.

(b) *Saddle synovial joint:* Between femur and patella.

Q. What are the articular surfaces in knee joint?

Ans. (a) Condyles of femur,

(b) Condyles of tibia and

(c) Patella.

Q. What are the bony landmarks in the region of the knee?

Ans.
1. *Adductor tubercle:* is felt just above the medial condyle of the femur.
2. *Head of the fibula:* is felt at posterolateral aspect of the knee. Lies 1.5 cm below the level of the knee joint.
3. *Tibial tubercle:* is felt in front of the knee in upper part of the tibia.
4. *Tibial condyles:* are felt on each side of the lower part of the ligamentum patellae.

Q. Name the ligaments of knee joint.

Ans.
1. Fibrous capsule
2. Ligamentum patellae
3. *Collateral ligaments:*Tibial and Fibular
4. *Popliteal ligaments:* Oblique and Arcuate
5. *Cruciate ligaments:* Anterior and Posterior
6. *Meniscus:* Medial and Lateral
7. Transverse ligament.

Q. What is coronary ligament?

Ans. It is the part of fibrous capsule lying between the menisci and tibia.

Q. What are the openings in the fibrous capsule of knee joint?

Ans.
1. For suprapatellar bursa and
2. For the exit of tendon of popliteus with its synovial bursa.

Q. What are the attachments of arcuate popliteal ligament?

Ans. It passes from the head of fibula to the posterior margin of the intercondylar area of tibia.

Q. What are the attachments of oblique popliteal ligament?

Ans. It arises as an expansion from the tendon of semimembranous. It blends with the posterior surface of fibrous capsule.It is attached to the intercondylar line and lateral condyle of femur and posterior aspect of medial condyle of tibia.

Q. Name the structures piercing oblique popliteal ligament?

Ans.
1. Posterior division of obturator nerve and
2. Middle genicular nerve and vessels.

Q. What are menisci and what the their functions?

Ans. These are two fibrocartilaginous structures, semilunar in shape, which make the tibial articular surface deeper.and divide the joint cavity partially into upper and lower compartment.

Functions:

(a) They act as shock absorbers.

(b) They make the articular surfaces more congruent. They can adapt to varying curvatures of different parts of femoral condyles.

Q. What is the arterial supply of knee joint?

Ans.
1. Genicular branches of popliteal artery,
2. Descending genicular branch of femoral artery,
3. Descending branch of lateral circumflex femoral artery.

4. Recurrent branches of anterior tibial artery and
5. Circumflex fibular branch of posterior tibial artery.

Q. Name the arteries forming the anastomosis around the knee joint.

Ans. *Medially:*

(i) Descending genicular
(ii) Superior medial genicular
(iii) Inferior medial genicular

Laterally:

(i) Descending branch of lateral circumflex femoral
(ii) Superior lateral genicular
(iii) Inferior lateral genicular
(iv) Anterior lateral recurrent
(v) Posterior lateral recurrent
(vi) Circumflex fibular.

Q. What is the nerve supply of knee joint?

Ans. 1. Femoral nerve,
2. Genicular branches of tibial and common peroneal nerves and
3. Posterior division of obturator nerve.

Q. What are the movements possible at knee joint?

Ans. 1. Flexion
2. Extension
3. Medial and lateral rotation.

Q. What is 'conjunct' and 'adjunct' rotation?

Ans. 1. *Conjunct rotation:* Rotation of knee joint combined with flexion and extension.
2. *Adjunct rotation:* Rotation of knee joint occurring independently in a partially flexed knee.

Q. What are the changes in the axis of movement of the knee joint with flexion and extension?

Ans. The flexion and extension of the knee joint takes place on a transverse axis which shifts along with the movements. Because of the spiral profiles of the femoral condyles, the axis shifts upwards and forwards during extension and backwards and downwards during flexion.

Q. What are the locking and unlocking movements of the knee joint?

Ans. In full extension from the position of flexion the last 30° of extension is accompanied by medial rotation of the femur on the tibia or lateral rotation of the tibia on the femur depending on whether the tibia or the femur is fixed. This is conjunct rotation and occurs passively as a part of the extension movement, is described as 'locking' of the knee joint.

From the position of full extension, the beginning of flexion is accompanied by lateral rotation of the femur or medial rotation of the tibia depending on whether the tibia or the femur is fixed. This rotation is called 'unlocking' of the knee joint. The contraction of popliteus is responsible for this unlocking movement.

Q. Name the intra-articular structures of the knee joint.

Ans.
1. *Cruciate ligaments:* Anterior and posterior
2. *Menisci:* Medial and lateral
3. Infrapatellar pad of fat
4. Synovial membrane
5. Origin of popliteus.

Q. Name the bursa around knee joint?

Ans. *Anteriorly:*
1. Subcutaneous prepatellar bursa
2. Subcutaneous infrapatellar bursa
3. Deep infrapatellar bursa and
4. Suprapatellar bursa.

Medially;
1. Bursa deep to medial head of gastrocnemius.
2. Bursa deep to tibial collateral ligament.
3. Semimembranosus bursa
4. Anserine bursa and
5. Occasionally, bursa between tendons of semitendinosus and semimembranosus.

Laterally:
1. Bursa deep to lateral head of gastrocnemius
2. Bursa between fibular collateral ligament and tendon of popliteus
3. Bursa between fibular collateral ligament and biceps femoris and

4. Bursa between tendon of popliteus and lateral condyle of tibia.

Q. Name the bursa communicating with the knee joint.

Ans. 1. Suprapatellar bursa
2. Popliteal bursa
3. Bursa deep to medial head of gastrocnemius.

Q. What is Anserine bursa?

Ans. It is bursa with several diverticula which separate the tendons of sartorius, gracilis and semitendinosus from bony surface of tibia.

Q. Name the different muscles producing movements of knee joint.

Ans.

	Principal muscles	*Accessory muscles*
(a) Extension	Quadriceps femoris	Tensor fasciae lata
(b) Flexion	Semitendinosus, Biceps femoris, Semimembranosus.	Sartorius, Gracilis, Popliteus, Gastrocnemius.
(c) Medial rotation	Semitendinosus, Semimembranosus.	Sartorius, Gracilis.
(d) Lateral rotation	Biceps femoris.	

Q. Name ligaments which become taut in full extension and flexion of the knee joint.

Ans. (a) *In full extension:*
(i) Anterior cruciate ligament.
(ii) Tibial and fibular collateral ligament.
(iii) Oblique popliteal ligament.
(b) *In full flexion:*
Posterior cruciate ligament.

Q. What could cause a tear of the menisci (semilunar cartilages) of the knee joint?

Ans. The menisci are usually torn by a twisting force with knee flexed. When the flexed knee is forcibly abducted and externally rotated, the medial meniscus is trapped between the medial condyles of the femur and tibia and is torn.

A severe adduction and internal rotation of the flexed knee may result in a tear of the lateral meniscus. But this injury is less common.

Q. Why the tears of medial meniscus are more frequent than that of lateral meniscus?

Ans. Because the medial meniscus is more firmly attached to the upper surface of the tibia, capsule and the tibial collateral ligament and therefore, is less able to adapt itself to sudden changes of position. The lateral meniscus on the other hand, is drawn backwards and downwards on the groove on the posterior aspect of the lateral tibial condyle by the medial fibres of popliteus. This prevents, the lateral meniscus from being impacted between the articular surfaces of the femur and the tibia during movements of the knee joint.

Q. Why in tear of medial meniscus there is locking of the knee before it is fully extended?

Ans. Because the torn segment of the cartilage is displaced and lodges between the femoral and tibial condyles and prevents full extension of the knee.

Q. Why the pain of hip joint is referred to the knee?

Ans. Because of the common nerve supply of the two joints.

ANKLE JOINT

Q. What type of joint is ankle joint?

Ans. Hinge variety of synovial joint.

Q. What are the articular surface of ankle joint?

Ans. *From above:*

1. Lower end of tibia with medial malleolus
2. Lateral malleolus and
3. Inferior transverse tibiofibular ligament.

From below: Body of talus.

Q. Name the ligaments of ankle joint.

Ans. (a) Fibrous capsule

(b) *Lateral ligament:* Consists of

1. Anterior talofibular ligament,
2. Posterior talofibular ligament and
3. Calcaneofibular ligament.

(c) *Medial (Deltoid) ligament:* It has

1. *Superficial part:* Consists of
   (i) Anterior fibres (Tibionavicular)
   (ii) Middle fibres (Tibiocalcanean) and
   (iii) Posterior fibres (Posterior tibiotalar).
2. *Deep part* (Anterior tibiotalar).

Q. Name the tendons crossing the deltoid ligament.

Ans. (i) Tibialis posterior and
(ii) Flexor digitorum longus.

Q. Name the structures related to ankle joint.

Ans. *Anteriorly:* From medial to lateral side:
(a) Tibialis anterior.
(b) Extensor hallucis longus,
(c) Anterior tibial vessels,
(d) Deep peroneal nerve,
(e) Extensor digitorum longus and
(f) Peroneus tertius.

Posteriorly: From medial to lateral side
(a) Tibialis posterior,
(b) Flexor digitorum longus,
(c) Posterior tibial vessels,
(d) Tibial nerve,
(e) Flexor hallucis longus
(f) Peroneus brevis and
(g) Peroneus longus.

Q. What are the movements produced at ankle joint?

Ans. 1. Dorsiflexon
2. Plantar flexion
3. *Accessory movements:* With plantar flexion, slight amount of side to side gliding, abduction and adduction are permitted.

Q. What is the axis of movements of the ankle joint?

Ans. It is represented by a transverse line drawn across the front of the ankle about 1.25 cm above the tip of the medial malleolus.

Q. What is the close-pack position of the ankle joint?

Ans. Dorsiflexion is the close-pack position of the joint in which the wider front part of the talus articulates with the mortise formed by the malleoli and lower end of the tibia. In this position, there is maximal congruence of the joint surface and tension of the ligaments.

Q. Name the muscles producing movements at ankle joint.

Ans. (a) *Dorsiflexon:*

Main muscle: Tibialis anterior.

Accessory muscles:

(a) Externsor digitorum longus,
(b) Extensor hallucis longus and
(c) Peroneus tertius.

(b) *Plantar flexion:*

Main muscles:

(a) Gastrocnemius and
(b) Soleus

Accessory muscles:

(a) Flexor digitorum longus,
(b) Flexor hallucis longus,
(c) Tibialis posterior and
(d) Plantaris.

Q. What is most frequent fracture at the ankle joint?

Ans. Pott's fracture, usually produced by an abduction external rotation injury.

TIBIOFIBULAR JOINTS

Q. What type of joints are tibiofibular joints?

Ans. 1. *Superior tibiofibular joint:* Plane synovial joint.
2. *Lower tibiofibular joint:* Syndesmosis type of fibrous joint.

Q. Name the structures passing through interosseous membrane of tibiofibular joint.

Ans. 1. Anterior tibial vessles
2. Perforating branch of peroneal artery.

JOINTS OF FOOT

Q. What do you understand by inversion and eversion of foot?

Ans. *Inversion:* Movement in which medial border of foot is elevated and sole faces medially and inwards.

Eversion: Movement in which lateral border of foot is elevated and sole faces laterally and outwards.

Q. Name the joints at which inversion and eversion takes place.

Ans. 1. Subtalar (Talocalcanean) joint and
2. Talocalcaneonavicular joint.

Q. What is the axis of the inversion and eversion?

Ans. Oblique axis which runs forwards, upwards and medially.
It passes between back of calcaneum, sinus tarsi and superomedial aspect of neck of talus.

Q. Name the evertors of foot.

Ans. Mainly by, peroneus brevis and longus.
Also by, peroneus tertius.

Q. Name the invertors of foot.

Ans. *Principal muscles:*
(a) Tibialis anterior and
(b) Tibialis posterior.
Accessory muscles:
(a) Flexor hallucis longus and
(b) Flexor digitorum longus

Q. Why are the movements of inversion and eversion required in man?

Ans. Inversion and eversion of the foot are essential for walking on rough, uneven or sloping surfaces.

ARCHES OF FOOT

Q. Classify the arches of foot.

Ans. (a) Longitudinal arches: Two
1. Medial and
2. Lateral
(b) Transverse arch.

Q. How the arches of foot are maintained?

Ans. 1. By the configuration of articulating bones forming the arch.

2. By the ligaments and muscles binding the adjacent bones and ends of an arch.
3. By tendons of muscle which act as sling and thus help to suspend the arch from above.
4. Plantar aponeurosis by connecting anterior and posterior ends of longitudinal arches like a tie beam.

Q. What are the functions of arches of foot?

Ans. 1. Rigid support for the weight of body in standing position.
2. As mobile spring board during walking and running.
3. As shock absorbers in jumping.
4. Protects the soft tissues of sole of foot.

Q. How the medial longitudinal arch is formed?

Ans. By calcaneum, talus, three cuneiforms and three medial metatarsals. The summit of arch is formed by talus.

Q. How the lateral longitudinal arch is formed?

Ans. By the calcaneum, cuboid and lateral two metatarsals.

Q. How the transverse arch is formed?

Ans. By the bases of the five metatarsals and the adjancet cuboid and cuneiforms of both feet.

Q. What are the attachments of spring ligament?

Ans. It passes from anterior magin of sustentaculum tali of calcaneus to plantar surface of navicular bone.

Q. What are the attachments of long plantar ligament?

Ans. It is attached posteriorly to plantar surface of calcaneus in front of lateral and medial tubercles and anteriorly to plantar surface of cuboid distal to groove for peroneus longus.

Q. Which structures maintain the medial longitudinal arch?

Ans. (a) The bony configuration do not contribute to the maintenance of this arch.

(b) *Ligaments:*

(i) The medial part of the plantar aponeurosis acts as a tie beam.

(ii) The plantar calcaneonavicular ('spring') ligament supports head of talus and forms intersegmental ties (connect adjacent bones).

(c) *Muscles:*

(i) Medial half of the flexor digitorum brevis and abductor hallucis act as tie beams (connect ends of arch).

(ii) Tibialis anterior, tibialis posterior and flexor hallucis longus act by forming sling and suspend the arch.

Q. How the lateral longitudinal arch of the food is maintained?

Ans. (a) *Ligaments:*

(i) The short plantar ligament, long plantar ligament and dorsal ligaments form intersegmental ties.

(ii) Lateral part of the plantar aponeurosis acts as a tie beam.

(b) *Muscles:*

(i) The peroneus longus and peroneus brevis muscles form the slings.

(ii) Lateral half of the flexor digitorum brevis and abductor digiti minimi act as tie beam.

Q. How the transverse arch of the foot is maintained?

Ans. (a) Tarsal and metatarsal bones contribute in maintaining the concavity of arch.

(b) *Ligaments*

(i) Ligaments that bind together the cuneiforms and the bases of the metatarsals form intersegmental ties.

(ii) Superficial and deep transverse metatarsal ligaments act as tie beams.

(v) *Muscles:*

(i) The peroneus longus and tibialis posterior form slings.

(ii) Abductor hallucis acts as tie beam.

Q. What are the deformities of the foot resulting from defects of the longitudinal arches of the foot?

Ans. 1. *Pes planus* (Flat foot): Due to flattening of the longitudinal arch, in particular the medial arch.

2. *Pes cavus* (High arched foot): The congenital form is probably due to shortness of the plantar fascia (apcneurosis). The acquired form can be due to contracture of the intrinsic muscles of the foot.

Q. What is the 'talipes deformity' of the foot?

Ans. In talipes the foot no longer lies in the plantigrade position. The person walks either on the heels or on the toes. When he walks on the heel the condition is known as *talipes calcaneus* while walking on the toes is known as *talipes equinus.* In both these conditions the foot may be inverted (*varus*) or everted (*valgus*).

Q. What is Hallus valugs?

Ans. In hallux valugs, there is lateral deviation of the great toe at the metatarsophalangeal joint. More common in women than men.

Q. What is 'Hammer toe'?

Ans. The affected toe is hyperextended at metatarsophalangeal and distal interphalangeal joint and flexed at proximal interphalangeal joint.

THIGH

Q. What is midinguinal point and what is its importance?

Ans. Midinguinal point is a point midway between anterior superior iliac spine and the pubic symphysis. It is an important land mark. The femoral artery and head of femur lie beneath the midinguinal point.

Q. What is Holden's line and what is its importance?

Ans. The deep layer of superficial fascia is firmly attached to the deep fascia of thigh along an horizontal line a little lateral to pubic tubercle and extends for about 8 cm laterally. This line of firm attachment is called Holden's line.

Clinical Importance: The extravasation of urine between these two layers cannot extend into thigh because of the firm attachment.

Q. How is patellar plexus formed?

Ans. It is a plexus of nerves in front of patella and upper end of tibia. It is formed by

(i) Anterior division of lateral and medial cutaneous nerve of thigh
(ii) Intermediate cutaneous nerve of thigh and
(iii) Infrapatellar branch of saphenous nerve.

Q. What is Housemaid's knee?

Ans. Chronic enlargement of prepatellar bursa is known as Housemaid's knee because it commonly occurs in housemaid's who have to kneel regularly for sweeping the floor.

Q. What is Miner's beat knee?

Ans. It is acute suppurative prepatellar bursitis in miners.

Q. What is Clergyman's knee?

Ans. It is enlargement of subcutaneous infrapatellar bursa in clergyman.

Q. What is Iliotibial tract and what are its functions?

Ans. The thickening of fascia lata on the lateral side of the thigh is called the iliotibial tract.

Functions:

1. Iliotibial tract stabilizes knee both in extension and partial flexion, *i.e.*, during walking and running.
2. In leaning forwards with slightly flexed knees, it is the only antigravity force to support the knee.

Q. What are the modifications of deep fascia of thigh?

Ans. (a) *Saphenous opening:*

Oval gap 4 cm below and lateral to pubic tubercle. Upper, lateral and lower margins form a crescentic sharp edge and medially deep part of fascia passes behind the femoral sheath.

(b) *Cribriform fascia:*

Cover the saphenous opening and is pierced by great saphenous vein, two superficial arteries and lymphatics.

(c) *Iliotibial tract:*

Receives insertion of ¾ of gluteus maximus and tensor fasciae latae.

FEMORAL TRIANGLE

Q. Why femoral triangle is known as Scarpa's triangle?

Ans. Because it was first described by Antonio Scarpa (1747-1832) in Italy.

Q. What are the boundaries of femoral triangle?

Ans. It is bounded by

Laterally: Medial border of sartorius.

Medially: Medial border of adductor longus.

Base: Inguinal ligament.

Apex: Directed downwards and is formed by meeting of medial and lateral boundaries.

Roof:

(a) Skin,

(b) Superficial fascia and

(c) Deep fascia.

Floor:

(a) Laterally by iliacus and psoas major.

(b) Medially by adductor longus and pectineus.

Q. What are the contents of femoral triangle?

Ans.

1. Femoral artery,
2. Branches of femoral artery:
   (a) Deep branches: Profunda femoris, deep external pudendal, descending genicular, saphenous and muscular.
   (b) Superficial branches: Superficial external pudendal, superficial epigastric and superficial circumflex iliac.
3. Femoral vein (medial to artery) and its tributaries
4. Femoral sheath
5. Femoral nerve (lateral to artery)
6. Nerve to pectineus
7. Femoral branch of genitofemoral nerve
8. Lateral cutaneous nerve of thigh and
9. Deep inguinal lymph nodes.

Q. What is Femoral sheath?

Ans. It is a funnel shaped fascial sleeve enclosing the upper 1½ inches of the femoral vessels.

Q. How is femoral sheath formed?

Ans. It is formed by the downward extension of the abdominal fasciae. The anterior wall is formed by fascia transversalis and posterior wall by fascia iliaca.

Q. What are the relations of femoral sheath?

Ans. *Anterior:*

(a) Skin
(b) Superficial fascia and
(c) Deep fascia with saphenous opening and great saphenous vein.

Posterior:

(a) Iliopectineal fascia
(b) Pectineus and
(c) Iliopsoas.

Lateral:

(a) Femoral nerve and
(b) Iliacus.

Medial:

(a) Lacunar ligament
(b) Pectineus and
(c) Pubic bones.

Q. What are the parts of femoral sheath?

Ans. The cavity within femoral sheath is divisible in three parts. Lateral part contains femoral artery and femoral branch of genitofemoral nerve. Middle part contains femoral vein and medial part is called femoral canal.

Q. What is femoral canal?

Ans. It is the medial compartment of the femoral sheath. It is conical and ½ inch wide at base and ½ inch long.

Q. What is femoral ring?

Ans. The base or upper end of the femoral canal is called the femoral ring.

The femoral ring is filled by condensed extraperitoneal tissue, the *femoral septum*, containing a lymph node and covered by parietal peritoneum.

Q. What are the boundaries of the femoral ring?

Ans. *Anterior:* Inguinal ligament.

Posterior: Pectineus and its fascia.

Lateral: Septum separating it from the femoral vein.
Medial: Concave margin of lacunar ligament.

Q. What are the contents of femoral canal?

Ans. (i) Lymph node (of Cloquet or of Rosenmuller).
(ii) Lymphatics.
(iii) Areolar tissue.

Q. What are the functions of femoral canal?

Ans. 1. It serves as a dead space for expansion of the femoral vein.
2. It allows a lymphatic pathway from the lower limb to the external iliac lymph nodes.

Q. What structure is drained by lymph node of femoral canal?

Ans. Glans penis in the male and clitoris in female.

Q. What is the clinical importance of the femoral canal?

Ans. The femoral canal is a potential point of weakness in the lower abdominal wall through which a viscus (intestines or urinary bladder) may protrude and give rise to a femoral hernia.

Q. Why is a femoral hernia commoner in females?

Ans. Because the femoral canal is larger in the females due to the greater width of the pelvis and smaller size of the femoral vessels. In the females, there is a rise in intra-abdominal pressure due to pregnancy predisposing to femoral hernia.

Q. Why is strangulation more common in femoral hernia?

Ans. Because the neck of the femoral canal is narrow.

Q. What is the risk of enlarging the opening of the femoral canal in releasing the strangulation of a femoral hernia?

Ans. In order to enlarge the opening of the femoral canal the sharp lateral edge of the lacunar (Gimbernat's) ligament may require incision. An abnormal obtuator artery may occasionally be present, which passes behind the lacunar ligament and is then in danger of being cut.

Q. What are the coverings of femoral hernia?

Ans. From within outwards:

(a) Peritoneum
(b) Femoral septum
(c) Femoral sheath
(d) Cribriform fascia
(e) Superficial fascia
(f) Skin.

ADDUCTOR CANAL

Q. What are the boundaries of the adductor canal?

Ans. *Posteriorly:*

(a) Adductor longus above and
(b) Adductor magnus below.

Anteriorly: Vastus medialis.

Medially: Sartorius which lies on a fascial sheet extending across the anterior and posterior walls.

Q. What is the extent of the adductor canal?

Ans. It extends from the apex of the femoral traingle to the tendinous opening in the adductor magnus.

Q. What are the contents of the adductor canal?

Ans.

1. Femoral artery.
2. Femoral vein.
3. Descending genicular branch of the femoral artery.
4. Saphenous nerve.
5. Nerve to vastus medialis.
6. Obturator nerve.

POPLITEAL FOSSA

Q. What are the boundaries of the popliteal fossa?

Ans. *Superolaterally:* Biceps femoris tendon.

Superomedially: Semimembranosus and Semitendinosus.

Inferomedially: Medial head of gastrocnemius.

Inferolaterally: Lateral head of gastrocnemius and Plantaris.

Q. Which structures form the floor of the popliteal fossa?

Ans. From above downwards:
1. The popliteal surface of the femur
2. The capsule of the knee joint
3. Popliteal fascia.

Q. What is the relationship between the tibial nerve and popliteal vessels in the popliteal fossa?

Ans. From superficial to deep lie, the tibial nerve, popliteal vein and popliteal artery. The popliteal artery is crossed by the popliteal vein and tibial nerve posteriorly from the lateral to medial side.

Q. What are the contents of popliteal fossa?

Ans.
1. Popliteal artery and its branches.
2. Popliteal vein and its tributaries.
3. Tibial nerve and its branches.
4. Common peroneal nerve and its branches.
5. Genicular branch of obturator nerve.
6. Posterior cutaneous nerve of thigh.
7. Popliteal lymph nodes.
8. Fat.

GLUTEAL REGION

Q. Name the structures passing through greater sciatic foramen.

Ans. (a) Piriformis

(b) Structures passing above piriformis
1. Superior gluteal nerve
2. Superior gluteal vessels

(c) Structures passing below piriformis
1. Inferior gluteal vessels
2. Internal pudendal vessels
3. Inferior gluteal nerve
4. Sciatic nerve
5. Posterior cutaneous nerve of thigh
6. Nerve to quadratus femoris
7. Pudendal nerve
8. Nerve to obturator internus.

Q. Name the structures passing through lesser sciatic foramen.

Ans. (a) Tendon of obturator internus
(b) Internal pudendal vessels
(c) Pudendal nerve
(d) Nerve to obturator internus.

Q. Name the structures lying under cover of gluteus minimus.

Ans. (a) Reflected head of rectus femoris
(b) Capsule of hip joint.

Q. What are the structures lying under cover of gluteus medius?

Ans. (a) Superior gluteal nerve
(b) Deep branch of superior gluteal artery
(c) Gluteus minimus
(d) Trochanteric bursa of gluteus medius.

Q. Name the structures lying under the cover of gluteus maximus

Ans. *(a) Ligaments*

1. Sacrotuberous
2. Sacrospinous and
3. Ischiofemoral

(b) Bones and joints

1. Ilium
2. Ischium with ischial tuberosity
3. Upper end of femur with greater trochanter
4. Sacrum
5. Coccyx
6. Hip joint
7. Sacroiliac joint.

(c) Bursae

1. Trochanteric bursa of gluteus maximus
2. Bursa over ischial tuberosity and
3. Bursa between gluteus maximus and vastus lateralis.

(d) Muscles

1. Gluteus medius
2. Gluteus minimus
3. Reflected head of rectus femoris

4. Piriformis
5. Obturator internus
6. Superior and inferior gemelli
7. Quadratus femoris
8. Obturator externus
9. Origin of hamstrings
10. Insertion of adductor magnus.

(e) Vessels

1. Superior gluteal vessels
2. Inferior gluteal vessels
3. Internal pudendal vessels
4. Ascending branch of medial circumflex femoral artery
5. Trochanteric anastomosis
6. Cruciate anastomosis
7. First perforating artery.

(f) Nerves

1. Superior gluteal ($L_{4,5}$ S_1)
2. Inferior gluteal (L_5, $S_{1,2}$)
3. Sciatic ($L_{4,5}$ $S_{1,2,3}$)
4. Posterior cutaneous nerve of thigh ($S_{1,2,3}$)
5. Nerve to quadratus femoris ($L_{4,5}$ S_1)
6. Pudendal nerve ($S_{2,3,4}$)
7. Nerve to obturator internus (L_5, $S_{1,2}$)
8. Perforating cutaneous nerve ($S_{2,3}$).

Q. What is Waddling gait?

Ans. Results from bilateral paralysis of gluteus medius and minimus so that the patient walks with swaying to clear the feet off the ground. When unilateral then it is known as *lurching gait*.

LEG AND FOOT

Q. Name the bony prominences felt in the leg and foot.

Ans. 1. Medial and lateral condyles of tibia.

2. *Tibial tuberosity:* In front of upper part of tibia, 2.5 cm below the line passing between tibia condyles.
3. *Head of fibula:* Posterolaterally at level of tibial tuberosity.

4. Anterior border and medial surface of tibia.
5. *Medial malleolus of tibia:* On medial side of ankle.
6. Lateral malleolus of fibula.
7. *Peroneal trochlea:* About a finger breadth below lateral malleolus.
8. *Sustentaculum tali:* About a finger breadth below medial malleolus.
9. *Tuberosity of navicular bone:* 2.5 to 3.5 cm antero-inferior to medial malleolus.
10. *Tuberosity of base of fifth metatarsal:* On lateral border of foot.

Q. What are the parts of deep fascia of leg?

Ans. (a) *Intermuscular septa:*

1. *Anterior and posterior intermuscular septa:* Divide leg into three compartments anteriors, lateral and posterior.
2. *Superficial transverse fascial septum:* Separates superficial and deep muscles of back of leg. Also forms flexor retinacula.
3. *Deep transverse fascial septum:* Separates tibialis posterior from long flexors of toes.

(b) *Retinacula:*

(i) *Extensor retinacula:* Superior and inferior.
(ii) *Peroneal retinacula:* Superior and inferior.

Q. What are the attachment of inferior extensor retinacula?

Ans. It is a Y-shaped retinacula.

Stem: Attached to anterior and articular part of superior surface of calcaneum.

Upper band: Attached to anterior border of medial malleolus

Lower band: Attached to plantar aponeurosis.

Q. Name the structures passing deep to inferior extensor retinacula.

Ans. (a) Tibialis anterior
(b) Extensor hallucis longus
(c) Deep peroneal nerve
(d) Anterior tibial vessels.

Q. Name the muscles of posterior compartment of leg.

Ans. *Superficial muscles:*

(a) Gastrocnemius,
(b) Soleus and
(c) Plantaris.

Deep muscles:

(a) Popliteus,
(b) Flexor digitorum longus,
(c) Flexor hallucis longus and
(d) Tibialis posterior.

Q. Name the structures passing under the flexor retinaculum.

Ans. From medial to lateral and above downwards are:

(a) Tibialis posterior tendon
b. Flexor digitorum longus tendon
c. Posterior tibial vessels
d. Tibial nerve
e. Flexor hallucis longus tendon.

Q. What is Tendocalcaneus?

Ans. It is a long tendon, receiving the insertion of fibres of soleus, gastrocnemius, both medial and lateral head.

Q. What is the insertion of tibialis anterior?

Ans. Tibialis anterior is inserted into medial side of medial cuneiform and base of first metatarsal.

Q. Where is peroneus longus inserted?

Ans. It is inserted into lateral side of medial cuneiform and base of first metatarsal

Q. Name the muscles found in different layers of sole of foot.

Ans. *From without inwards:*

First layer:

(a) Flexor digitorum brevis
(b) Abductor hallucis
(c) Abductor digit minimi.

Second layer:

(a) Flexor digitorum accessorius
(b) Lumbricals: Four in number

Third layer:

(a) Flexor hallucis brevis

(b) Flexor digiti minimi brevis

(c) Adductor hallucis

Fourth layer: Three plantar and four dorsal interossei.

Q. What is plantar aponeurosis and what are its functions?

Ans. It is the thickened central part of the deep fascia of sole.

Functions:

1. Provides attachment to skin of sole.
2. Gives origin to muscles of first layer of sole.
3. Protects the digital vessels and nerves and deeper muscles.
4. Helps in maintaining the longitudinal arch of the foot.

Q. What are the functions of interossei of sole?

Ans. (a) *Dorsal interossei:* Abductors of the toes.

(b) *Plantar interossei:* Adductors of the toes.

ARTERIAL SUPPLY OF LOWER LIMB

Q. What is the extent of femoral artery?

Ans. It begins at mid inguinal point and ends at medial side of middle and lower one third of thigh by passing through an aperature in adductor magnus muscle to reach back of thigh and become popliteal artery.

Q. Name the branches of profunda femoris.

Ans. (a) Lateral circumflex femoral artery

(b) Medial circumflex femoral artery

(c) Perforating arteries

(d) Muscular branches

Q. Name the arteries forming the cruciate anastomosis.

Ans. (a) Inferior gluteal artery

(b) First perforating artery

(c) Transverse branch of medial circumflex femoral artery

(d) Transverse branch of lateral circumflex femoral artery.

Q. Name the arteries forming the trochanteric anastomosis.

Ans. (a) Descending branch of superior gluteal artery

(b) Ascending branch of medial circumflex femoral artery

(c) Ascending branch of lateral circumflex femoral artery.

Q. How the circulation is maintained in case of blockage of femoral artery?

Ans. In blockage in proximal part, circulation is maintained through cruciate and trochanteric anastomosis. When blockage is in lower thigh then circulation is maintained. through perforating branches of profunda femoris artery and its anastomoses with branches of the popliteal artery.

Q. Name the branches of popliteal artery.

Ans. (a) Cutaneous branches

(b) *Superior muscular branches:* To adductor magnus and hamstrings

(c) *Sural arteries:* To gastrocnemius, soleus and plantaris.

(d) *Superior genicular arteries:* Medial and lateral

(e) Middle genicular artery

(f) *Inferior genicular arteries:* Medial and lateral

(g) *Terminal branches:* Anterior and posterior tibial.

Q. What are the relations of anterior tibial artery in anterior compartment of leg?

Ans. (a) *Relation to muscles:* In upper 1/3, lies between tibialis anterior and extensor digitorum longus. In middle 1/3, lies between tibialis anterior and extensor hallucis longus. In lower 1/3, lies between extensor hallucis longus and extensor digitorum longus.

(b) *To veins:* Artery is accompanied by two venae comites.

(c) *To nerve:* Deep peroneal nerve is lateral to it in upper 1/3 and lower 1/3 and anterior to it in middle 1/3.

Q. What are the branches of anterior tibial artery?

Ans. 1. Muscular branches.
2. *Recurrent branches:* Anterior and posterior tibial
3. *Malleolar branches:* Anterior medial and anterior lateral.

Q. How dorsalis pedis artery is formed?

Ans. It is the continuation of anterior tibial artery in front of ankle between the two malleoli.

Q. Name the branches of dorsalis pedis artery.

Ans. 1. Lateral tarsal artery
2. Medial tarsal artery
3. Arcuate artery
4. First dorsal metatarsal artery.

Q. Where the pulsations of dorsalis pedis artery are felt?

Ans. Between the tendon of extensor hallucis longus and first tendon of extensor digitorum longus on dorsum of foot about 5 cm distal to medial and lateral malleoli, over intermediate cuneiform bone.

Q. Name the branches of posterior tibial artery.

Ans. 1. Peroneal: Largest branch
2. Muscular
3. Nutrient artery to tibia
4. *Anastomotic branches:*
   (a) Circumflex fibular
   (b) Communicating branch to peroneal
   (c) Malleolar
   (d) Calcaneal
5. *Terminal branches:* Medial and lateral plantar.

Q. To which bone peroneal artery gives a nutrient artery?

Ans. Fibula

Q. Which artery forms the plantar arch?

Ans. Lateral plantar artery

Q. How the lateral plantar artery terminates?

Ans. It ends by joining termination of dorsalis pedis artery in interval between bases of first and second metatarsal bone.

Also see Ch. Femoral triangle and Popliteal fossa.

VENOUS DRAINAGE

Q. What are the different factors which facilitate the return of venous blood to heart?

Ans. I. *Local factors:*

(a) Veins of lower limb are larger than veins of other parts of body. They also have greater number of valves, which prevent the back flow of blood.

(b) Muscular contraction, compresses the deep veins and drives the blood upwards.

(c) Muscular compression of veins is made more effective by tight deep fascia.

II. *General factors:*

(a) The valves which maintain a unidirectional flow.

(b) Negative intrathoracic pressure, which pulls the column of blood up and it is made more negative during inspiration.

(c) Vis-a-tergo (compulsion from behind) produced by arterial pressure and over flow from capillary bed.

Q. What are the main superficial veins of lower limb?

Ans. (a) *Great saphenous vein:* Continuation of medial marginal vein of foot. It ascends into thigh and after passing through saphenous opening in deep fascia ends in femoral vein. It receives superficial epigastric, superficial circumflex iliac, external pudendal, anterior vein of leg and posterior arch veins.

(b) *Anterior cutaneous vein of thigh:* Drains front of lower part of thigh and it drains into great saphenous vein.

(c) *Short saphenous vein:* Continuation of lateral marginal vein of foot and ends in popliteal vein above knee joint.

(d) *Perforating veins:* These are the veins connecting superficial veins with the deep veins after perforating the deep fascia. They permit only unidirectional flow of blood, from superficial to deep veins by means of valves. These are present both in thigh and leg, but a number of these are present in lower one third of leg.

Q. What is 'calf pump' or 'peripheral heart'?

Ans. In upright position, venous return from lower limb depends largely on the contraction of calf muscles, these are known as calf pump, the soleus is called "peripheral heart" for same reason.

Q. What are varicose veins?

Ans. If the valves in veins become incompetent, the pressure during muscular contraction is transmitted from deep veins to the superficial veins and hence, leakage of blood. This causes dilatation of the superficial veins, known as varicose veins. Later on gradual degeneration occurs, leading to "varicose ulcers".

Q. What is the clinical importance of sural sinuses?

Ans. Sural sinuses are the common site for thrombosis and commonly leads to pulmonary embolism due to the detachment of thrombus.

LYMPHATIC DRAINAGE OF LOWER LIMB

Q. What is the lymphatic drainage of various inguinal lymph nodes?

Ans. (a) *Upper lateral superficial group:* Drains skin of anterior abdominal wall below umbilicus.

(b) *Upper medial superficial group:* Drains skin of anterior abdominal wall below umbilicus, external genitalia except glans penis or clitoris, lower part of anal canal and lower part of vagina and some lymphatics from inguinal canal.

(c) *Lower superficial inguinal group:* Drains superficial lymphatics of lower limb except from back of leg.

(d) *Deep inguinal group:* Drains deep lymphatics of thigh, glans penis or clitoris and popliteal lymph nodes.

(e) *Popliteal lymph nodes:* Drains deep lymphatics of foot and leg and superficial lymphatics of back of leg.

All lymphatics from inguinal nodes drain into external iliac lymph nodes.

NERVES OF LOWER LIMB

LUMBAR PLEXUS

Q. How lumbar plexus is formed?

Ans. By the ventral rami L_{1-3} and greater part of ventral ramus of L_4. The first lumbar nerve also receives a branch from T_{12} nerve.

Q. What are the branches of lumbar plexus?

Ans. (a) *Muscular:*
To quadratus lumborum (T_{12}, L_{1-3})
Psoas minor (L_1)
Psoas major ($L_{2,3}$)
Iliacus ($L_{2,3}$)
(b) Iliohypogastric nerve (L_1)
(c) Ilioinguinal nerve (L_1)
(d) Genitofemoral nerve ($L_{1,2}$)
(e) Lateral cutaneous nerve of thigh (Dorsal division of ventral primary rami of $L_{2,3}$)
(f) Femoral nerve (Dorsal division of ventral primary rami of L_{2-4})
(g) Obtorator (Ventral division of ventral primary rami of L_{2-4})
(h) Accessory obturator (Ventral division of ventral primary rami of $L_{3,4}$).

Q. What is the distribution of obturator nerve?

Ans. (a) *Anterior branch* supplies:
1. *Muscular branches*: To adductor longus, gracilis, obturator externus and occasionally adductor brevis and pectineus.
2. *Articular*: To hip joint.
3. *Cutaneous*: To subsartorial plexus
4. *Vascular branches*: To femoral artery

(b) *Posterior branch* supplies:
1. *Muscular branches:* To obturator externus, adductor magnus and adductor brevis.
2. *Articular:* To knee joint.

Q. Name the branches of femoral nerve.

Ans. A. *Anterior division* supplies:

(a) Nerve to pectineus
(b) Intermediate cutaneous nerve of thigh
(c) Medial cutaneous nerve of thigh
(d) Nerve to sartorius
(e) Nerve to liliacus

B. *Posterior division* supplies:

(a) Saphenous nerve
(b) Muscular branches to quadriceps femoris
(c) Vascular branches to femoral artery
(d) Articular branches to hip and knee joint

Q. Name the nerves forming the subsatorial plexus.

Ans. (a) Medial cutaneous nerve of thigh
(b) Saphenous nerve
(c) Cutaneous branch of anterior division of obturator nerve.

Q. Name the nerves forming the pateller plexus.

Ans. (a) Saphenous nerve
(b) Medial, intermediate and lateral cutaneous nerve of thigh
(c) Saphenous nerve and its infrapatellaer branch

Q. What is 'meralgia paraesthetica'?

Ans. It is a clinical condition characterised by pain, tingling, numbness or anaesthesia in the area of distribution of the lateral cutaneous nerve of the thigh. This nerve (a branch of the lumbar plexus) usually enters the thigh, passing deep to the inguinal ligament. Occasionally, the nerve pierces the ligament and may then be compressed by it with resultant irritation of the nerve.

Q. What is the adductor spasm?

Ans. It is spasm of the adductor muscles of the thigh and occurs in spastic paraplegia.

Q. How can the pain of the adductor spasm be relieved?

Ans. By division of the obturator nerve.

Q. Why does a patient sometimes complain of pain in the knee when the disease is actually in the hip joint?

Ans. This is referred pain because both the hip and knee joints are supplied by the same nerves, i.e., the femoral and obturator nerves.

SACRAL PLEXUS

Q. How sacral plexus is formed?

Ans. By ventral primary rami of $L_{4,5}$ S_{1-4}.

Q. What are the branches of sacral plexus?

Ans. (a) Sciatic nerve ($L_{4,5}$ S_{1-3})
(b) Superior gluteal nerve (Posterior division of $L_{4,5}$ S_1)
(c) Inferior gluteal nerve (Posterior division of L_5, $S_{1,2}$)
(d) Perforating cutaneous nerve (Posterior division of $S_{2,3}$)
(e) Nerve to piriforenis (Posterior division of $S_{1,2}$)
(f) Pudendal nerve (Anterior division of S_{1-3})
(g) Posterior cutaneous nerve of thigh (Anterior division of $S_{1,2}$ and posterior division of $S_{2,3}$)
(h) Nerve to obturator internus (Anterior division of L_5, $S_{1,2}$)
(i) Nerve to quadratus femoris (Anterior division fo $L_{4,5}$ S_1)
(j) Nerve to levator ani and coccygeus and sphincter ani externus from S_4 branches
(k) Pelvic splanchnic nerve from S_{2-4}

Q. How the sciatic nerve is formed? What are its branches?

Ans. The sciatic nerve is the continuation of the sacral plexus and derives its fibers from the $L_{4,5}$, $S_{1,2,3}$. It is the largest nerve in the body. The main trunk of the sciatic nerve is the nerve of the flexor compartment of the thigh.

Branches:

(a) *Articular:* To hip joint.

(b) *Muscular:* To biceps femoris, semitendinosus, semimembranosus and ischial head of adductor magnus.

(c) Terminal:

i. The *tibial nerve* is the nerve of the flexor compartments of the thigh (through the parent trunk), leg and sole of the foot. It receives fibres from the anterior divisions of $L_{4,5}$ $S_{1,2}$ and S_3 (which does not divide into anterior and posterior division)

ii. The *common peroneal nerve* is the nerve of the extensor and peroneal compartments of the leg and dorsum of the foot. It is derived from the posterior divisions of $L_{4,5}$ $S_{1,2}$.

Q. Give the surface marking of the sciatic nerve.

Ans. The sciatic nerve is represented by a thick line (2 cm broad) joining the following three points.

The *first point* is taken 2.5 cm lateral to the mid-point of a line joining the posterior superior illiac spine (marked by a dimple lateral to the natal cleft) and the ischial tuberosity.

The *second point* is taken at the mid-point between the greater trochantar of the femur and the ischial tuberosity.

The *third point* is taken at the mid-point of a transverse line drawn at the junction of the middle and lower 2/3 of the back of the thigh, *i.e.*, apex of the popliteal fossa.

Q. What will be the effect of a complete lesion of the sciatic nerve in the gluteal region?

Ans. A. *Motor loss:*

i. Loss of flexion of the knee due to paralysis of the hamstring muscles, but some weak movement is possible due to the action of the sartorius (femoral nerve) and gracilis (obturator nerve).

ii. Loss of all movements below the knee due to paralysis of all the muscles of the leg and foot. There will be a *'foot drop'* deformity.

iii. Loss of achilles jerk and plantar reflex.

B. *Sensory loss:* On the outer side of the leg and almost the entire foot.

Q. What is 'sciatica' and what is its common cause?

Ans. Sciatica is the term applied when pain is felt along the course and distribution of the sciatic nerve, i.e., in the buttock, posterior aspect of the thigh and leg and lateral aspect of the leg and foot This is due to irritation of one or more of the roots of the sciatic nerve and commonly occurs due to a prolapsed intervertebral disc in the lumbar region.

Q. At what site intramuscular injections are given in gluteal region?

Ans. The injections are given in upper and outer quadrant of the gluteal region to avoid injury to the sciatic nerve.

Q. What is the site for local anaesthetic to be injected for sciatica to relieve the pain?

Ans. The site of injection is midway between the greater trochanter of the femur and the ischial tuberosity.

Q. What are the branches of common peroneal nerve?

Ans. (a) Lateral cutaneous nerve of calf

(b) Communicating branch to sural nerve

(c) Terminal branches: Deep and superficial peroneal nerve.

Q. Where is the common peroneal (lateral popliteal) nerve commonly injured and what are the common causes of the injury?

Ans. The nerve is commonly injured where it winds round the neck of the fibula. It may be damaged at this site by the pressure of a tight bandage of plaster cast, in severe adduction injury to the knee or from direct trauma.

Q. What will be the effects of a complete section of the common peroneal (lateral popliteal) nerve at the level of the neck of the fibula?

Ans. A. *Motor loss:*

i. Inability to extend the foot or toes due to paralysis of the ankle and foot extensors (tibialis anterior, extensor hallucis longus, extensor digitorum longus, peroneus tertius and extensor digitorum brevis). This results in "foot drop" which is characteristic of the common peroneal nerve injury.

ii. Inability to evert the foot due to paralysis of the peroneal muscles.

Paralysis of the extensor and evertor muscles of the foot causes the foot to assume a position of *equino-varus* (equinus: plantar flexion, varus: inversion), results in a slapping or high steppage gait (the patient-raises the knee high and the foot hangs flexed and inverted).

B. *Sensory loss:* Over the anterior and lateral aspects of the leg and foot. The lateral border of the foot and the lateral side of the little toe are unaffected since they are supplied by the sural branch of the tibial nerve.

Q. What are the structures supplied by deep peroneal nerve?

Ans. 1. *Muscular branches: To*

(a) Tibialis anterior
(b) Extensor hallucis longus
(c) Extensor digitorum longus
(d) Peroneus tertius and
(e) Extensor digitorum brevis

2. *Cutaneous branches:* To adjacent sides of first and second toes on dorsum of foot.
3. *Articular branches:* To ankle joint, tarsal and metatarsal joints.

Q. What is the effect of lesion of deep peroneal nerve?

Ans. *Sensory loss:* Adjacent sides' of I and II toe.

Motor loss: Paralysis of muscles supplied by it. So over activity of peroneal and flexor muscles leads to *Talipes equinovalgus*.

Q. Name the branches of superficial peroneal nerve.

Ans. 1. *Muscular branches:* To peroneus longus and peroneous brevis.

2. *Cutaneous branches:* To lower 1/3 of lateral side of leg and dorsum of foot supplying medial side of I toe, lateral side of II toe and III, IV, V toes.
3. *Communicating branches:* To sural, deep peroneal and saphenous nerve.

Q. What will occur if nerve supply to peroneal muscles is cut off?

Ans. Talipes varus.

Q. What is the distribution of tibial nerve?

Ans. (a) *Muscular branches* to gastrocnemius plantaris, soleus, popliteus, tibialis posterior, flexor digitorum longus, flexor hallucis longus.

(b) *Cutaneuos branches:*
Sural nerve
Medial calcaneal branch

(c) *Articular branches:* To knee and ankle joint

(d) *Terminal branches:* Medial and lateral plantar nerves

Q. What is the distribution of medial plantar nerve?

Ans. (a) *Cutaneous branches:*

1. From trunk, skin to medial part of sole
2. Skin on medial side of great toe
3. Three plantar digital nerves to medial 3½ digits

(b) *Muscular branches:*

1. From trunk to abductor hallucis and flexor digitorum brevis.
2. From digital nerve to great toe to flexor hallucis brevis
3. From first plantar digital nerve to first lumbrital

(c) *Articular branches:*

1. Tarsal and tarsometatarsal joints from main trunk
2. Metatarsophalangeal and interphalangeal joints from digital nerves.

Q. What is the distribution of lateral plantar nerve?

Ans. (a) *Cutaneous branches:*

1. From trunk to skin of lateral part of sole
2. Digital branches to lateral 1½ toes.

(b) *Muscular branches:*

1. From trunk to flexor digitorum accessorius and abductor digiti minimi.
2. Digital branch to lateral side of fifth toe supplies flexor digiti minimi, 3rd plantar and 4th dorsal interossei
3. Deep branch to adductor hallucis, 2nd, 3rd and 4th lumbricals, all interossi except above.

Q. Where is the tibial (medial popliteal) nerve commonly injured what are the common causes of the injury?

Ans. The tibial nerve may be damaged in or below the popliteal fossa by automobile accident, fractures of leg or by gunshot or stab wounds. The frequency of injuries to the tibial nerve is far less than the common peroneal nerve because of its deeper position and more protected course.

Q. What will be the effects of a complete section of the tibial (medial popliteal) nerve in the popliteal fossa?

Ans. A. *Motor loss:*

i. Inability to fully flex the ankle joint due to paralysis of the gastocnemius and soleus. A small degree of flexion is possible by the peroneus longus (which is supplied by the superficial peroneal nerve).

ii. Inability to invert the foot against resistance due to paralysis of the tibialis posterior.
The foot assumes the position of a *calcaneo-valgus* (calcaneus: dorsiflexion, valgus: eversion) by the unopposed action of the extensors and evertors. The patient cannot stand on tip-toe. Walking is difficult due to difficulty in 'taking off.

iii. Inability to flex the toes due to paralysis of both the long and short flexors of the toes.

iv. Ankle jerk is absent.

B. *Sensory loss* over the sole (except the inner border).

C. *Vasomotor and trophic changes* are common. The foot becomes oedematous, discoloured and cold. Trophic ulcers are almost inevitable.

Q. What is the cutaneous nerve supply of back of leg?

Ans. (a) *Saphenous nerve* ($L_{3,4}$): Branch of posterior division of femoral nerve. Supplies skin of medial area of leg and medial border of foot upto ball of I toe.

(b) *Posterior division of medial cutaneous nerve of thigh* ($L_{2,3}$): Supplies upper most part of medial area of calf.

(c) *Posterior cutaneous nerve of thigh* ($S_{1,2,3}$): Supplies upper ½ of central area of calf.

(d) *Sural nerve* (L_5,$S_{1,2}$): Branch of tibial nerve. Supplies lower ½ of central area and lower 1/3 of lateral area of calf and lateral border of foot.

(e) *Lateral cutaneous nerve of calf* ($L_{4,5}$ S_1): Branch of common peroneal nerve. Supplies skin of upper 2/3 of lateral area of leg.

(f) *Peroneal (Sural) communicating nerve* ($L_5S_{1,2}$): Branch of common peroneal nerve. Supplies skin of lateral area of calf.

(g) *Medial calcanean branches* ($S_{1,2}$): Supplies skin of heel and medial side of sole of foot.

Thorax

THORACIC CAGE

Q. How thoracic cage is formed?

Ans. *Anteriorly:* Sternum

Posteriorly: Twelve thoracic vertebrae and intervertebral discs

One each side: Twelve ribs with their cartilages.

Q. What variations occur in thorax with age?

Ans. (a) In adults, in transverse section thorax is reniform, with a greater transverse diameter than antero-posterior. In infants, circular in transverse section.

(b) In adults, ribs are oblique. In infants, ribs are horizontal.

Q. What are the boundaries of 'thoracic inlet'?

Ans. *Anteriorly:* Upper border of manubrium sterni.

Posteriorly: Upper border of body of T_1 vertebra.

One each side: First rib with its cartilage.

Q. What is the direction of plane of inlet of thorax?

Ans. Downwards and forwards with a obliquity of about 45 degrees. The upper border of manubrium sterni lies at level of upper border of T_3 vertebra.

Q. What is Sinson's fascia and what are its attachments?

Ans. It is a triangular membrane at thoracic inlet (Diaphragm of inlet of thorax).

Attachments:

Apex: Tip of transverse process of C_7 vertebra.

Base: laser border of first rib and its cartilage.

Inferior surface: Fused with cervical pleura.

Q. Name the structures passing through thoracic inlet.

Ans. *Muscles:*

(a) Sternohyoid

(b) Sternothyroid and
c) Longus colli.

Arteries:

(a) Right and left internal thoracic arteries
b) Brachiocephalic artery
(c) Left common carotid
d) Left subclavian and
(e) Right and left superior intercostal arteries.

Nerves:

(a) Left recurrent laryngeal nerve
(b) Right and left phrenic nerve
(c) Right and left vagus nerve
(d) Right and left first thoracic nerve and
(e) Right and left sympathetic chain.

Veins:

(a) Right and left brachiocephalic Vein
(b) Right and left posterior intercostal vein and
(c) Inferior thyroid veins.

Others:

(a) Thymus
(b) Trachea
(c) Oesophagus
(d) Anterior longitudinal ligament
(e) Right and left pleura and
f) Apex of right and left lung.

Q. What are the boundaries of outlet of thorax?

Ans. *Anteriorly:* Infrasternal (Subcostal) angle between two costal margins.

Posteriorly: Inferior surface of body of 12th thoracic vertebra.

On each side:

(a) Costal margin formed by 7th, 8th, 9th and 10th ribs and
(b) 11th and 12th ribs.

RIBS

Q. What are 'True ribs'?

Ans. First seven ribs connected through costal cartilages to sternum are called true ribs.

Q. What are 'false ribs'?

Ans. Last five ribs are known as false ribs.

Cartilages of 8th, 9th and 10th ribs are joined to each other and form *costal margin.*

Anterior ends of 11th and 12th ribs are free and are called *'floating ribs'*.

Q. What are typical and atypical ribs?

Ans. First two and last three ribs are called atypical because they present special features. The 3rd to 9th ribs are called typical because they have common features.

Q. What are the features of a typical rib?

Ans. Each typical rib has

1. *Anterior end:* Oval and articulates with costal cartilage.
2. *Posterior end:* It is made up of:
   (a) *Head:* Has two articular facets for articulation with vertebrae.
   (b) *Neck:* Has anterior and posterior surfaces and superior and inferior borders.
   (c) *Tubercle:* Medial part is articular.
3. *Shaft:* Has outer and inner surfaces and upper and lower borders.

Q. What are the relations of head of typical rib?

Ans. (a) Sympathetic chain and
(b) Costal pleura.

Q. What is costal groove? Name the structures attached and lying with in the costal groove?

Ans. Costal groove is a depression present between inferior border and ridge on inner surface.

Attachments: Origin of internal intercostal muscle from floor of groove.

Contents: From above downwards:

(a) Intercostal vein
(b) Intercostal artery and
(c) Intercostal nerve.

Q. What are the special features of 1st rib?

Ans. 1. It is flattened from above downwards.
2. It is shortest, broadest and most curved rib.

3. Twist at angle of shaft is absent.
4. Head has one articular facet.
5. It has no costal groove.

Q. Name the structures related to neck of first rib.

Ans. *Anteriorly* from medial to lateral side:

(a) Sympathetic trunk with cervicothoracic ganglion
(b) First posterior intercostal vein
(c) Superior intercostal artery and
(d) First thoracic nerve.

Superiorly:

(a) Deep cervical vessels and
(b) C_8 nerve.

Q. What are the structures related to grooves on superior surface of first rib?

Ans. (a) *Anterior groove:* Subclavian vein.
(b) *Posterior groove:* Subclavian artery and Lower trunk of brachial plexus.

Q. What is the difference in ossification of 1st and other typical ribs?

Ans. The typical ribs have three secondary centres, one for head and two for tubercle.

The first rib has two secondary centres, one for head and one for tubercle.

Q. What are the special features of 2nd, 10th, 11th and 12th rib?

Ans. *Second rib:*

(a) Sharply curved like first rib
(b) Shaft has no twist
(c) Outer surface of shaft has a rough tubercle
(d) Inner surface faces more downwards.

Tenth rib:

(a) Shorter than typical rib
(b) Single facet on head.

Eleventh rib:

(a) Short
(b) Neck and tubercle absent
(c) Anterior end pointed
(d) Angle slight
(e) Groove shallow.

Twelth rib:

(a) Short
(b) Neck and tubercle absent
(c) Anterior end pointed
(d) Angle absent
(e) Groove absent-

Q. In which rib both superior and inferior costotransverse ligaments are absent?

Ans. 12th rib.

Q. What is the characteristic of cortovertebral joint of 1st, 10th, 11th and 12th ribs?

Ans. These ribs articulate only with corresponding vertebrae.

Q. What is the commonest site of rib fracture in adults?

Ans. The rib is fractured at the angle, which is its weakest point.

Q. Why the fracture of ribs are rare in children?

Ans. Because in the children the chest wall is highly elastic.

Q. What is 'Stove in chest'?

Ans. This is produced in severe crush injuries in which multiple rib fractures are produced along with permanent indentation of chest wall.

Q. What is 'Flail chest'?

Ans. This results from more severe injury to chest. Multiple rib fractures at two or more sites result in unstable chest wall in which flail area is sucked inwards during inspiration and pushed out in expiration.

Q. What is cervical rib?

Ans. (a) Present in 0.5% of cases.
(b) It is attached to the transverse process of 7th cervical vertebra and its distal extremity is free or articulates with first thoracic rib.

Q. What is the clinical importance of a cervical rib?

Ans. It may press on the lower trunk of brachical plexus producing paraesthesiae along ulnar border of forearm and wasting of small muscles of hand. Less commonly, vascular changes are produced due to .pressure on subclavian artery.

Q. What is the histological structure of costal cartilage?

Ans. It is made up of hyaline cartilage.

Q. What type or joints costal cartilage form?

Ans. (a) *With the rib and manubrium:* Primary cartilaginous joint:
(b) *With the sternum:* Synovial joint.
(c) 8th to 10th cartilages medially are connected to each other.

STERNUM

Q. What are the parts of sternum?

Ans. (a) Manubrium
(b) Body and
(c) Xiphoid process.

Q. What is Jugular notch?

Ans. Also called suprasternal notch, present in middle of superior border of manubrium.

Q. What is the level of jugular notch?

Ans. It lies at level of intervertebral disc between T_2 and T_3 vertebra.

Q. What is sternal angle (Angle of Louis)?

Ans. It is the angle formed at the junction of manubrium and body of sternum. It is convex forwards.

Q. What is the level of sternal angle?

Ans. Intervertebral disc between T_4 and T_5 vertebra.

Q. What is the clinical significance of sternal angle?

Ans. It is an important landmark for counting ribs as 2nd costal cartilages articulates with sternum of this level.

Q. Name the structures lying at level of sternal angle.

Ans. (a) Ascending aorta ends.
(b) Arch of aorta begins and also ends.

(c) Descending aorta begins.
(d) Pulmonary trunk divides into two pulmonary arteries.
(e) Marks the upper limit of base of heart.
(f) Azygous vein opens into superior vena cava.
(g) Trachea divides into two principal bronchi.

Q. Why the sternum is commonly used for getting a specimen of bone marrow?

Ans. Because cortical bone of sternum is very thin and subcutaneous. It is therefore easily accessible.

Q. What types of joints are present between different parts of sternum?

Ans. *Between manubrium and body (Manubriosternal joint):* Secondary cartilaginous joint.
Between body and xiphisternum (Xiphisternal joint): Primary cartilaginous joint.

Q. Which rib is attached to junction of body with xiphoid process?

Ans. Seventh costal cartilage

Q. What type of joint is sternocostal joint?

Ans. Synovial joint

Q. What is the level of Xiphisternal joint?

Ans. 9th thoracic vertebra.

Q. What is 'Funnel chest'?

Ans. Deformity of chest in which the body of sternum and xiphoid process is depressed. This predisposes to respiratory and cardiovascular disturbances.

Q. What is 'Pigeon chest'?

Ans. It is condition in which deformity of chest occurs due to forward projection of sternum and flattening of chest on either side.

Q. What is 'Ectopia cordis'?

Ans. In this, the sternum and adjoining parts of costal cartilages and ribs are missing. So that the heart can be seen from outside.

THORACIC VERTEBRAE

Q. What are the typical' and 'atypical' thoracic vertebrae?

Ans. *Typical thoracic vertebrae:* 2nd to 8th, they have common features.

Atypical vertebrae: 1st, 9th to 12th, they have special features.

Q. What are the structures attached to transverse process?

Ans.
1. *Lateral costotransverse ligament:* At tip.
2. *Inferior costotransverse ligament:* On anterior surface.
3. *Superior costotransverse ligament:* On lower border.
4. *Intertransverse muscles:* Upper and lower borders.
5. *Levatorcostae:* To posterior surface.

Q. What is the characteristic feature of a typical thoracic vertebrae?

Ans. It has costal facets on sides of vertebral bodies and transverse processes for articulation with ribs.

Q. What movement is possible in the thoracic spine?

Ans. Rotation, greater in lower thoracic region as compared to upper thoracic region.

INTERCOSTAL SPACES

Q. What are intercostal spaces?

Ans. Gaps between ribs and their costal cartilages are called intercostal spaces.

Q. What are typical intercostal spaces?

Ans. The 3rd to 8th spaces are typical intercostal spaces. The blood and nerve supply of 3rd to 6th intercostal space is limited only to the thoracic while those of lower spaces extend into the abdomen.

Q. What are the contents of a typical intercostal space.

Ans. (a) *Muscles:*

i. External intercostal

ii. Internal intercostal and
iii. Transversus thoracis (Innermost intercostal).

(b) Intercostal nerve

(c) Intercostal vessels and lymphatics.

Q. What is the attachment and extent of external intercostal muscle?

Ans. (a) *Attachment:*

Origin: Lower border of the rib above.

Insertion: Outer lip of the upper border of the rib below.

Fibres run downward, and medially in anterior part and downwards and laterally in posterior part.

(b) *Extent:* From the tubercle of rib behind to its costochondral junction in front where it continues as external intercostal membrane.

Q. What is the attachment and extent of internal intercostal muscle?

Ans. (a) *Attachment:*

Origin: Floor of the costal groove of the rib above.

Insertion: Inner lip of the upper border of the rib below. Fibres are at right angles to those of external intercostal.

(b) *Extent:* From the lateral margin of the sternum to the angle of the rib where it continues as the internal intercostal membrane.

Q. Name the muscles which comprise the transversus thoracic group of muscles.

Ans.
1. Subcostalis
2. Intercostalis intimi and
3. Sternocostalis.

Q. What is the attachment of muscles comprising transversus thoracic group of muscles?

Ans. They form the innermost layer of the muscles of the thoracic wall.

1. *Subcostalis:* Present in posterior parts of the lower spaces. They are attached to the inner surface of rib near angle and to the inner surface of the second or third rib below.

2. *Intercostalis intimi:* Present in the middle 2/4 of the upper spaces, except in the 1st space. They arise from inner surface of the upper rib and are inserted into the inner surface of the rib below.
3. *Sternocostalis:* Present in the anterior part of the upper spaces, except in the 1st space. They arise from the lower part of the posterior surface of the body of the sternum and the xiphoid process and the adjacent costal cartilages (4th to 7th). They pass upwards and laterally and are inserted by slips to the costal cartilages of the 2nd to 6th ribs-

   The direction of fibres of these three parts is same as internal intercostal muscle.

Q. What is the position of neurovascular plane of thorax?

Ans. Between internal intercostal muscle and intercostalis intimi and posteriorly between pleura and internal intercostal membrane. The vein is highest, artery is in middle and nerve is lowest.

Q. What will happen if intercostal muscles are paralysed?

Ans. There will a retraction of intercostal spaces during inspiration and bulging during expiration.

Q. How intercostal nerves are formed and how they are distributed?

Ans. These are the ventral primary rami of T_1- T_{11} nerves. The ventral primary rami of T_{12} forms subcostal nerve.

T_1 and T_2 supply the upper limb.

T_3 to T_6 supply thoracic wall (Typical intercostal nerves).

T_7 to T_{11} supply abdominal wall.

Q. What are the branches of a typical intercostal nerve?

Ans. 1. *Communicating:*

(a) White ramus communicans
(b) Grey ramus communicans
} Connected to sympathetic ganglion.

2. *Muscular:*

(a) *Muscular branches:* Supplies intercostal muscles, serratus posterior superior.

(b) *Collateral branch:* Supplies intercostal muscles, parietal pleura and periosteum of rib.

3. *Cutaneous:*
   (a) *Lateral cutaneous branch:* Emerges at mid axillary line. Divides into anterior and posterior branches.
   (b) *Anterior cutaneous branch:* Emerges at lateral border of sternum.

Q. What is the characteristic feature of second thoracic nerve?

Ans. Its lateral cutaneous branch forms the *intercostobrachial nerve* which enters the upper limb and supplies the skin on medial side of upper arm.

Q. Where the pain due to irritation of intercostal nerves is referred to?

Ans. To the front of chest or abdomen, i.e., at the peripheral termination of nerve.

Q. What is the course of pus from vertebral column around the thorax?

Ans. The pus may track along the course of neurovascular bundle and may point at the exit of cutaneous branches of intercostal nerve, i.e., lateral to erector spinae, in mid axillary line and just lateral to the sternum.

Q. Name the arteries of intercostal space.

Ans.
1. One posterior intercostal artery and
2. Two anterior intercostal arteries.

Q. Name the branches of posterior intercostal arteries?

Ans.
(a) Dorsal branch
(b) Muscular branches
(c) Collateral intercostal branch
(d) Lateral cutaneous branch and
(e) *Mammary branches:* Of 2nd, 3rd, and 4th arteries.
(f) Right bronchial artery: From right third posterior intercostal artery.

Q. What is the origin of intercostal arteries?

Ans. (a) Posterior intercostal arteries:
1st and 2nd: From superior intercostal artery which is a branch of costocervical trunk.
3rd to 11th: From descending thoracic aorta.

(b) Anterior intercostal arteries:

Of 1st to 6th space: From internal thoracic artery, which is a branch of first part of subclavian artery.

Of 7th to 9th space: From musculophrenic artery, terminal branch of internal thoracic artery.

10th and 11th spaces don't have anterior intercostal arteries.

Q. How the intercostal veins terminate?

Ans. (a) *Anterior intercostal veins:* Two in each of upper nine spaces.

In upper six spaces: Drain into internal thoracic vein. *In lower three spaces:* Into musculophrenic vein.

(b) *Posterior intercostal vein:* One in each of eleven spaces. *Mode of termination is:*

On left side:

1st: Into left brachiocephalic vein.

2nd and 3rd: Form left superior intercostal vein which drains into left brachiocephalic vein.

4th to 8th: Into accessory hemiazygos vein.

9th to 11th and subcostal veins: Into hemiazygos vein.

On right side:

1st: Into right brachiocephalic vein.

2nd and 3rd: Form right superior intercostal vein which drains into azygos vein.

4th to 11th and subcostal vein: Into azygos vein.

Q. Name the branches of internal thoracic artery.

Ans. (a) Pericardiophrenic

(b) Mediastinal

(c) Anterior intercostals of upper six spaces

(d) Perforating

(e) Superior epigastric and

(f) Musculophrenic.

Q. What type of movement of ribs take place during the respiration?

Ans. The anterior end of ribs can move up during inspiration and down during expiration by rotation at costovertebral and costotransverse joints. This increases anteroposterior diameter of thorax. Angular movement at manubriosternal joint of upper six ribs leads to forward movement of ribs.

In inspiration, middle of rib is raised. This occurs at costotransverse and sternocostal joint at 7th to 10th ribs and increases transverse diameter of thorax. Elevation of ribs is produced by external intercostal and depression by internal intercostal during quiet breathing.

PLEURAE

Q. What is pleura?

Ans. It is a serous membrane, lined by mesothelium. There are two pleural sacs, one on either side of mediastinum.

Q. What are the parts of pleura?

Ans. *Outer layer:* Parietal pleura.

Inner layer: Visceral pleura.

The two layers are continuous with each other at the hilum of lung. The two layers enclose between them a potential space known as *pleural cavity*.

Q. What are the parts of parietal pleura?

Ans. (a) *Costal:* Lines the thoracic wall and is loosely attached to it by areolar tissue.

(b) *Diaphragmatic:* Lines upper surface of diaphragm.

(c) *Mediastinal:* Lines mediastinum.

(d) *Cervical:* Extends into neck and covers apex of lung. Covered by Sibson's fascia.

Q. What is the extent of cervical pleura in neck?

Ans. It extends two inches above the first costal cartilage and one inch above medial ½ of clavicle.

Q. What are the relations of cervical pleura?

Ans. *Anteriorly:* Subclavian artery and
Scalenus anterior muscle.

Posteriorly: Neck of first rib with its relations.

Medially: Large vessels of neck.

Laterally: Scalenus medius.

Q. What is 'Pulmonairy ligament'? What are its functions?

Ans. It is parietal pleura surrounding the root of lung which hangs down as a fold called pulmonary ligament.

Functions:

1. It provides dead space into which veins of lung can expand when venous return increases.
2. Because of it, lung root can descend with the descent of diaphragm.

Q. What are the 'recesses of pleura'?

Ans. These are folds of parietal pleura, which act as reserve spaces, into which lungs can expand during deep inspiration.

Three in number:

(a) *Costomediastinal recess:* Present in cardiac notch of left lung anteriorly, between costal and mediastinal pleurae.

(b) *Costodiaphragmatic recess:* On both sides inferiorly, between costal and diaphragmatic pleurae

Q. What are the parts of lung not covered with visceral pleura?

Ans. At hilum and along the attachment of pulmonary ligament where it is continuous with parietal pleura.

Q. What is the nerve supply of pleura?

Ans. (a) *Parietal pleura:* Pain sensitive.

Intercostal nerves: Costal and diaphragmatic pleurae at periphery.

Phrenic nerves: Mediastinal and central part of diaphragmatic pleurae.

(b) *Visceral pleura:*

Pain insensitive.

Sympathetic nerves (T_2-T_5).

Q. What is the arterial supply of pleura?

Ans. *Parietal pleura:* Intercostal arteries,
Internal thoracic arteries and
Musculophrenic arteries.

Visceral pleura: Bronchial arteries.

Q. What is the lymphatic drainage of pleura?

Ans. *Parietal pleura:* Lymphatics drain into intercostal, internal mammary, mediastinal and diaphragmatic lymph nodes.

Visceral pleura: Drained by bronchopulmonary lymph nodes.

Q. What is the developmental origin of pleura?

Ans. *Parietal pleura:* Somatopleural layer of lateral plate mesoderm.

Visceral pleura: Splanchnopleural layer of lateral plate mesoderm.

Q. What is the surface marking of pleura?

Ans. *Cervical pleura:* Curved line forming a dome over the medial 1/3 of clavicle. The apex of curve lies 2.5 cm. above the clavicle.

Anterior margin:

(a) *On right side:* From sternoclavicular joint downwards and medially to mid point of sternal angle, where it continues vertically downwards to mid point of xiphisternal joint.

(b) *On left side:* Same course upto fourth costal cartilage, where it arches and descends along sternal margin of 6th costal cartilage, about 3 cm from midline.

Inferior margin: Laterally from lower limit of anterior margin, so that it crosses the 8th rib in midclavicular line, 10th rib in mid axillary line and 12th rib at lateral border of sacrospinalis. Then horizontally to lower border of T_{12} vertebra, about 2 cm from midline.

Posterior margin: From a point 2 cm. lateral to 12th thoracic spine to a point 2 cm. lateral to 7th cervical spine.

Q. What are the places at which pleura descends below costal margin?

Ans.
1. Right costoxiphoid angle.
2. Right costovertebral angle below 12th rib.
3. Left costovertebral angle below 12th rib.

Q. What is Pneumothorax?

Ans. A pneumothorax is produced by the presence of air in the pleural cavity.

Q. What is haemothorax?
Ans. It is the blood in the pleural cavity.

Q. What is pleural effusion?
Ans. It is the accumulation of free fluid in the pleural cavity.

Q. What is empyema?
Ans. It is accumulation of pus in the pleural cavity.

Q. What is empyema necessitatis?
Ans. An abscess over thoracic wall secondary to collection of pus in pleural cavity.

Q. What is 'Paracentesis thoracis' and from which site it is done?
Ans. It is the process of aspiration of any fluid from the pleural cavity.
Done in 6th intercostal space in mid axillary line.

Q. What are the structures pierced during paracentesis?
Ans. The structures pierced from outward to inwards in midaxillary line are: Skin, fascia, serratus anterior muscle, intercostal muscles and parietal pleura to reach pleural cavity.

Q. What precaution should be taken during aspiration from pleural cavity?
Ans. Needle should be pricked in lower part of intercostal space to avoid injury to intercostal nerves and vessels in costal groove

Q. What is Meig's syndrome?
Ans. It is a triad of:
(a) Ovarian fibroma (benign tumour to ovary),
(b) Ascites (fluid in peritoneal cavity) and
(c) Right sided pleural effusion.

LOWER RESPIRATORY TRACT

TRACHEA

Q. What is the extent of trachea?
Ans. Trachea extends from 6th cervical vertebra (lower border of cricoid cartilage) to lower border of 4th thoracic vertebra where it divides into right and left bronchi.

Q. What are the relations of cervical part of trachea?

Ans. *Anteriorly:*

(a) Isthmus of thyroid gland,
(b) Inferior thyroid veins below isthmus,
(c) Anastomosis between left and right superior thyroid arteries
(d) Jugular arch
(e) Pretracheal fascia,
(f) Sternohyoid muscle,
(g) Sternothyroid muscle;
(h) Investing layer of deep cervical fascia,
(i) Superficial fascia and
(j) Skin.

Posteriorly:

(a) Oesophagus,
(b) Longus colli and
(c) Recurrent laryngeal nerve.

On each side:

(a) Thyroid gland,
(b) Common carotid artery and
(c) Inferior thyroid artery.

Q. What are the relations of thoracic part of trachea.

Ans. *Anterior:*

(a) Manubnum sterni,
(b) Sternothyroid and sternohyoid muscle,
(c) Thymus,
(d) Left brachiocephalic vein,
(e) Inferior thyroid vein,
(f) Aortic arch,
(g) Brachiocephalic artery,
(h) Left common carotid artery,
(i) Deep cardiac plexus and
(j) Lymph nodes.

Posterior:

(a) Oesophagus and
(b) Vertebral column.

Right side:

(a) Right pleura,
(b) Right lung,
(c) Right vagus,
(d) Azygous vein,

(e) Right brachiocephalic vein and
(f) Superior vena cava.

Left side:

(a) Arch of aorta,
(b) Left common carotid artery,
(c) Left subclavian artery and
(d) Left recurrent laryngeal nerve.

Q. What is the arterial supply of trachea?

Ans. Inferior thyroid arteries.

Q. What is the nerve supply of trachea?

Ans. *Parasympathetic nerves:* Vagus through recurrent laryngeal. It is

(a) Sensory } to mucous membrane
(b) Secretomotor } to mucous membrane
(c) Motor to tracheal muscle

Sympathetic nerves: Through middle cervical ganglion. It is vasomotor.

Q. What is the lymphatic drainage of trachea?

Ans. To

(a) Pretracheal lymph nodes and
(b) Paratracheal lymph nodes.

Q. What are the variations in the level of bifurcation of trachea with respiration?

Ans. *Bifurcation of trachea, normally:* Between T_4 and T_5 vertebra.

In deep inspiration: T_6 vertebra.

In expiration: T_4 vertebra.

Q. Where trachea can be palpated?

Ans. In suprasternal notch midway between sternal ends of two clavicles.

Q. What is 'Tracheal tug'?

Ans. Arch of aorta lies in close relation to trachea and left bronchus. In aneurysm of aortic arch, a pull or drag is felt on the trachea which is known as 'tracheal tug'.

Q. How the trachea appear in an X-ray?

Ans. Since trachea is more radiolucent (because of air in it) than neighbouring structures, it appears as a dark area passing downwards, backwards and slightly to the right.

Q. What are the common causes and effects of tracheal compression?

Ans. *Causes:* Pathological enlargement of surrounding structures especially thyroid gland and arch of aorta.
Effects: Dyspnoea, cough, husky voice.

Q. In what conditions the tracheostomy is done?

Ans. (a) In laryngeal obstruction.
(b) For removal of excessive secretions.
(c) For long continued artificial respiration.

Q. What is the commonest site for tracheostomy?

Ans. It is most commonly done in retrothyroid region after cutting the isthmus of thyroid gland. Usually the second and third tracheal rings are cut.

Q. Why the tracheostomy is difficult and dangerous in children?

Ans. Because
(a) Neck is relatively short and left innominate vein may come up above suprasternal notch.
(b) Trachea is softer and more mobile, so it is not readily identified and isolated.

Q. What is the histological structure of trachea?

Ans. Trachea consists of following layers from within outwards:
(a) *Mucosa:* Lined by pseudostratified columnar ciliated epithelium. Lamina propria has mainly reticular fibres.
(b) *Submucosa:* Loose areolar tissue.
(c) *Cartilages and muscles:* C-shaped hyaline cartilages make the framework of trachea.
Posterior gap has transverse fibres of smooth muscles and fibroelastic membrane.
(d) Adventitia.

Q. What is the advantage of posterior gap in tracheal cartilage?

Ans. Posteriorly, the oesophagus lies close to trachea so the oesophagus can dilate into posterior membranous part, during passage of food bolus.

BRONCHI

Q. What are the differences between right and left main bronchus?

Ans.

Right main bronchus	Left main bronchus
(a) Wider, shorter (2.5 cm) more vertical	Narrower, longer (5 cm) and less vertical.
(b) Passes to root of lung at T_5.	Passes to root of lung at T_6
(c) Divides into 3 lobar bronchi	Divides into 2 lobar bronchi.
(d) *Relations:*	
i. Azygos vein arches over it from behind to reach superior vena cava	i. It passes below the arch of aorta, in front of oesophagus and descending aorta
ii. Right pulmonary artery lies first below and then anterior to it.	ii. Left pulmonary artery lies first anterior and then above it.
iii. Right upper pulmonary vein covers right principal bronchus	iii. Left upper pulmonary vein crosses in front of the bronchus.

Q. Why the foreign bodies and aspirated material tend to pass into right bronchus rather that into left?

Ans. Because of the greater width and more vertical course of the right bronchus.

LUNGS

Q. What is a broncho-pulmonary segment?

Ans. The main bronchus on each side gives off branches to each lobe of the lung, *lobar bronchus*. Each lobar bronchus then divides into *segmental bronchi*, each of which supplies a segment of the lung called a *bronchopulmonary segment*. Each segmental bronchus is accompanied by a branch of the pulmonary artery and a tributary of the pulmonary vein. The arteries lie posterolateral to the corresponding bronchi. Pulmonary veins tend to run between adjacent bronchopulmonary segments, therefore each vein may drain **more** than one segment.

Each broncho-pulmonary segment is therefore a self contained, functionally independent respiratory unit of lung tissue.

These segments are wedge shaped with their apices at the hilum and bases at the lung surface. Each is surrounded by connective tissue continuous with that of the visceral pleura. There are also veins which run between the segments and are called intersegmental veins.

Q. Name the broncho-pulmonary segments of the two sides.

Ans. Each broncho-pulmonary segment receives its name from that of its supplying segmental bronchus.

Right side	Left side
Upper lobe	*Upper lobe*
1. Apical segment	1. } Apico-posterior
2. Posterior segment	2. } segment
3. Anterior segment	3. Anterior segment
Middle lobe	*Lingular*
4. Lateral segment	4. Superior segment
5. Medial segment	5. Inferior segment
Lower lobe	*Lower lobe*
6. Apical (superior) segment	6. Apical (superior) segment
7. Medial basal (cardiac) segment	7. Anterior basal segment
8. Anterior basal segment	8. Lateral basal segment
9. Lateral basal segment	9. Posterior basal segment
10. Posterior basal segment	

On the left side, the upper lobe bronchus gives off a combined apico-posterior segmental bronchus whereas on the right they arise separately as apical and posterior segmental bronchi.

The left upper lobe has a lingular segment which is equivalent to the right middle lobe.

On the right side there is a medial basal segmental bronchus which is absent on the left.

Q. Why the knowledge of the bronchial tree and broncho-pulmonary segments is important?

Ans. It is important:

1. During bronchoscopy
2. For correct interpretation of bronchograms
3. To determine the appropriate posture for promoting drainage of infected areas of lung
4. For surgical resection of a single or a number of diseased broncho-pulmonary segments without affecting the function of the remaining segments.

Q. What are the differentiating features of the two lungs?

Ans. 1. The right lung has three lobes while the left lung has two lobes.

2. The thin, sharp anterior border of the right lung is vertical while that of the left lung presents a cardiac notch.
3. On the medial surface (mediastinal surface) of the lung, the cardiac impression is much deeper on the left than on the right.
4. The right lung is wider than the left because of the smaller cardiac impression.
5. The right lung is shorter then the left because of the higher position of the right dome of the diaphragm.

Q. Name the structures in root of lungs.

Ans. 1. Principle bronchus on left side and eparterial and hyparterial bronchi on right side.

2. One pulmonary artery.
3. Superior and inferior pulmonary vein.
4. *Bronchial arteries:* One on right and two on left side.
5. Bronchial veins.
6. Anterior and posterior pulmonary plexuses of nerves.
7. Lymphatics of lung.
8. bronchopulmonary lymph nodes.
9. Areolar tissue.

Q. At what level the root of lungs lie?

Ans. Opposite body of T_{5-7} vertebra.

Q. What are the relations of the structures at the root of the lung?

Ans. From above downwards (differs on two sides)

Right lung	*Left lung*
1. Eparterial bronchus	1. Pulmonary artery
2. Pulmonary artery	2. Bronchus
3. Hyparterial bronchus	3. Inferior pulmonary vein
4. Inferior pulmonary vein	

From before backwards (similar on two sides):

1. Superior pulmonary vein,
2. Pulmonary artery and
3. Bronchus.

Q. What is the surface marking of the oblique fissure of the lung?

Ans. It corresponds approximately with the medial border of the scapula when the arm is raised above the shoulder.

The fissure may be represented by a line drawn obliquely from a point 2 cm, lateral to the 4th thoracic spine on the right side and at a slightly higher level on the left side to another point on the 5th rib in the midaxillary line and a third point on the 6th costal cartilage about 7.5 cm from midline.

Q. Where can the breath sound of the apical segment of the lower lobe be heard on auscultation?

Ans. Posteriorly below the upper end of the oblique fissure.

Q. Give the surface marking of the horizontal fissure of the right lung.

Ans. It corresponds approximately with a line drawn horizontally at the level of the 4th costal cartilage anteriorly. This line meets that of the oblique fissure in the mid axillary line.

Q. What is the 'lingula' of the left lung?

Ans. The upper lobe of the left lung corresponds with the upper and middle lobes of the right lung. The part of it which corresponds to the middle lobe is called the 'lingula' because it projects anteriorly to form the lingula (tongue-shaped structure) below the cardiac notch.

Q. What is the 'azgos lobe'?

Ans. The azygos vein is occasionally deeply embedded in the apex of the right lung, partly isolating its medial portion. This isolated medial portion of the right lung is referred to as the 'azygos lobe'.

Q. What is 'sequestration of lung'?

Ans. An area of lung not having any communication with the bronchial passages. Most frequently seen in lower lobe of left lung.

Q. What is the lymphatic drainage of the lung?

Ans. The lymphatics of the lung drain centripetally from the pleura towards the hilum into the broncho-pulmonary lymph nodes. Efferents of these nodes drain into the tracheo-bronchial nodes which drain into the *paratracheal nodes and the mediastinal lymph trunks.* These lymph trunks drain directly into the brachiocephalic vein, or occasionally, indirectly via the right lymphatic duct or the thoracic duct.

MEDIASTINUM

Q. Define mediastinum?

Ans. It is a median septum of thorax between two pleural cavities. Strictly speaking, it is septum between two lungs because mediastinal pleurae are also part of it.

Q. What are the boundaries of mediastinum?

Ans. *Superiorly:* Thoracic inlet
Inferiorly: Diaphragm
Anteriorly: Sternum
On each side: Mediastinal pleura.

Q. What are the divisions of mediastinum?

Ans. Mediastinum is divided by an imaginary plane passing anteriorly through sternal angle and posteriorly through T_4 vertebra into:

(a) Superior mediastinum
(b) *Inferior mediastinum:* Subdivided by pericardium into:

1. *Anterior mediastinum:* In front of pericardium
2. *Middle mediastinum:* Pericardium and its contents
3. *Posterior mediastinum:* Behind pericardium.

Q. What are the boundaries of superior mediastinum?

Ans. *Anteriorly:* Manubrium sterni

Posteriorly: Upper 4 thoracic vertebrae.

Superiorly: Plane of thoracic inlet.

Inferiorly: Imaginary plane between superior and inferior mediastinum.

On each side: Mediastinal pleura.

Q. Name the contents of superior mediastinum.

Ans. *Arteries:*

(a) Arch of aorta,
(b) Brachiocephalic artery,
(c) Left common carotid artery and
(d) Left subclavin artery.

Veins:

(a) Right and left brachiocephalic veins,
(b) Upper ½ of superior vena cava and
(c) Left superior intercostal vein.

Muscles: Origin of

(a) Sternothyroid,
(b) Sternohyoid and
(c) Longus colli.

Nerves:

(a) Phrenic,
(b) Vagus,
(c) Cardiac and
(d) Left recurrent laryngeal.

Lymph nodes and lymphoid tissue:

(a) Thymus
(b) Thoracic duct and
(c) Lymph nodes.

Tubes:

(a) Trachea and
(b) Oesophagus.

Q. What are the contents of anterior mediastinum?

Ans. (a) Superior and inferior sternopericardial ligaments,
(b) Lymph nodes,

(c) Mediastinal branches of internal thoracic artery,
(d) Areolar tissue and
(e) Thymus.

Q. What is the arterial supply of thymus?

Ans. The thymus is supplied by inferior thyroid and internal thoracic arteries

Q. What is the function of thymus?

Ans. Thymus is primary lymphoid organ and it play a vital role in making lymphocytes, immunologically competent T lymphocytes.

Q. Name the contents of middle mediastinum.

Ans. (a) Heart with pericardium
(b) Ascending aorta
(c) Pulmonary trunk
(d) Pulmonary arteries
(e) Bifurcation of trachea
(f) Principal bronchi
(g) Lower half of superior vena cava
(h) Terminal part of azygous vein
(i) Pulmonary veins
(j) Phrenic nerve
(k) Deep cardiac plexus and
(l) Tracheobronchial lymph nodes.

Q. What are the contents of posterior mediastinum?

Ans. (a) Descending thoracic aorta
(b) Azygous vein
(c) Hemiazygous vein
(d) Accessory hemiazygous vein
(e) Vagus nerves
(f) Greater splanchnic nerve
(g) Lesser splanchnic nerve
(h) Least splanchnic nerve
(i) Thoracic duct
(j) Posterior mediastinal lymph nodes and
(k) Oesophagus.

Q. What is mediastinal syndrome?

Ans. Compression of mediastinal structure by any growth gives rise to a group of symptoms known as mediastinal syndrome.

Q. How the pus in posterior mediastinum can enter the thighs?

Ans. The fascial sheath of psoas major muscle is open by its upper attachment to L_2 or L_1 vertebra. This upper edge forms medial lumbocostal arch, from which vertebral part of diaphragm arises. So, psoas sheath opens into posterior mediastinum by a funnel shaped orifice. Pus in posterior mediastinum enters through funnel shaped orifice and along the psoas sheath extends into thighs.

Q. Why the infection behind the prevertebral layer of deep cervical fascia cannot extend into posterior mediastinum?

Ans. The prevertebral layer of deep cervical fascia extends to the superior mediastinum and is attached to the 4th thoracic vertebra, so the neck infections behind this fascia can not extend down beyond T_4.

Q. Infections between which layers of cervical fascia can extend into posterior mediastinum?

Ans. Posterior mediastinum is continuous through superior mediastinum with the neck between pretracheal and prevertebral layers of cervical fascia.
This region includes retrophrayngeal space, spaces on each side of trachea and oesophagus, space between trachea and oesophagus.

PERICARDIUM

Q. What is pericardium?

Ans. It is a fibroserous sac enclosing the heart and roots of great vessels.

Q. What are the parts of pericardium?

Ans. (a) *Fibrous pericardium:* Outer, single layered, tough and fibrous.
(b) *Serous pericardium:* Inner, double layered, thin.

Q. What are the attachments of fibrous pericardium?

Ans. Fibrous pericardium is conical in shape.

Apex: Blunt and fused with roots of great vessels and pretracheal fascia.
Base: Blends with central tendon of diaphragm.
Anteriorly: By superior and inferior sternopericardial ligaments, attached to body of sternum.

Q. What are the different layers of serous pericardium?

Ans. (a) *Parietal pericardium:* Outer, fused with fibrous pericardium.
(b) *Visceral pericardium:* Inner, fused to heart except where it is separated from heart by blood vessels.

Both layers are continuous at root of great vessels.

Q. What is pericardial cavity?

Ans. It is a potential space between parietal and visceral layers. It contains a thin layer of serous fluid.

Q. What is oblique sinus of pericardium?

Ans. It is a space behind heart between the left atrium, anteriorly and parietal pericardium, inferiorly.

Q. What is transverse sinus of pericardium?

Ans. It is a horizontal gap between ascending aorta and pulmonary trunk anteriorly and superior vena cava and atrium posteriorly.
On each side it opens into pericardial cavity.

Q. What is surgical importance of transverse sinus?

Ans. Through this sinus a temporary ligature is given to occlude pulmonary trunk and aorta during cardiac operations.

Q. What is the developmental origin of sinuses of pericardium?

Ans. *Transverse sinus:* Develops due to degeneration of dorsal mesocardium.
Oblique sinus: Develops due to absorption of pulmonary veins into left atrium.

Q. What is the nerve supply of pericardium?

Ans. (a) *Fibrous and parietal pericardium:* By phrenic nerve. They are pain sensitive.
(b) *Visceral pericardium:* By autonomic nerves of heart.

Q. What is the arterial supply of pericardium?

Ans. (a) *Visceral layer:* By coronary arteries.

(b) *Fibrous and parietal layer:* By branches of internal thoracic, musculophrenic and descending thoracic aorta.

Q. What are the contents of the pericardium?

Ans. (i) Heart with cardiac vessels and nerves

(ii) Ascending aorta

(iii) Pulmonary trunk

(iv) Lower half of superior vena cava

(v) Terminal part of inferior vena cava and

(vi) Terminal part of pulmonary veins.

HEART

Q. What is the position of heart?

Ans. It is placed obliquely behind body of sternum and adjoining parts of costal cartilages of ribs.

1/3 of it lies to right and 2/3 of it lies to left of median plane.

Q. What are the divisions of heart?

Ans. Heart is composed of four chambers:

(a) Two atria: Right and left

(b) Two ventricles: Right and left.

The atria are separated from ventricles by *coronary sulcus* (atrioventricular groove).

The atria are separated by *interatrial groove* and the ventricles by *anterior and posterior interventricular grooves.*

Q. Name the structures in anterior and posterior interventricular grooves.

Ans. *In anterior interventricular groove:*

(a) Interventricular branch of left coronary artery and

(b) Great cardiac vein.

In posterior interventricular groove:

(a) Interventricular branch of right coronary artery and

(b) Middle cardiac vein.

Q. Which chambers form the upper border of heart?

Ans. Two atria, chiefly left atrium.

Q. Which chambers form the left border of heart?

Ans. Mainly by left ventricle and
Partly by left auricle.

Q. Name the chambers forming the surfaces of heart?

Ans. *Anterior surface:*
Mainly, by right ventricle and right auricle.
Partly, by left ventricle and left auricle.
Inferior surface:
Left 2/3 by left ventricle and
Right 1/3 by right ventricle.
Left surface:
Mostly by left ventricle and upper end by left auricle.
Posterior surface (Base):
Mainly by left atrium.
Small part by posterior part of right atrium.

Q. What is right auricular appendage and what are its characteristic features?

Ans. It is the upper prolonged end of right atrium, which covers the root of ascending aorta. Externally, it is notched and interior is sponge like.

Q. What is the clinical importance of structure of right auricular appendage?

Ans. Its sponge like interior prevents free flow of blood and favour thrombosis which may dislodge to cause pulmonary embolism.

Q. What are the parts of right atrium and how they are developed?

Ans. Three parts:
(a) *Smooth posterior part (Sinus venarum):* Derived from right horn of sinus venosus. All large veins entering right atrium open in this part.
(b) *Rough anterior part including auricle (Atrium proper):* Derived from primitive atrial chamber.
(c) *Septal wall:* Derived from septum primum and septum secondum.

Q. Name the veins opening in the right atrium?

Ans. (a) Superior vena cava,
(b) Inferior vena cava,
(c) Coronary sinus
(d) Anterior cardiac veins and
(e) Venae cordis minimi.

Q. What is Eustachian valve?

Ans. It is a rudimentary valve guarding the opening of inferior vena cava. During embryonic life it guides the inferior caval blood to left atrium through foramen ovale.

Q. What are the features of septal wall of right atrium?

Ans. It has
(a) *Fossa ovalis:* Saucer shaped depression in lower part, formed by septum primum.
(b) *Limbus fossae ovalis:* It is prominent margin of fossa ovalis and represents free edge of septum secondum.

Q. What are the parts of right ventricle?

Ans. (a) *Inflowing part:* Rough and has muscular ridges called *trabeculae carneae.*
(b) *Outflowing part:* Smooth. Also called infundibulum. Opens into pulmonary trunk.
The two parts are separated by a ridge, *supraventricular crest* and the inflow and outflow parts make an angle of about 90° with each other.

Q. What are the different types of trabeculae carneae?

Ans. (a) *Ridges:* Fixed elevations.
(b) *Bridges*: Fixed at ends but free in middle.
(c) *Papillary muscles:* Bases attached to ventricular wall and apex project into ventricular cavity and are connected to chordae tendineae.

Q. How the left atrium is developed?

Ans. (a) Greater part is smooth and is derived from absorption of pulmonary vein.
(b) Auricle develops from primitive atrial chamber.

Q. What are the parts of left ventricle?

Ans. *Out flow part:* Known as aortic vestibule. Opens into ascending aorta. Inflow part same as right ventricle. The inflow and outflow parts are at an acute angle.

Q. What is fossa lunata?

Ans. It is an impression in septal wall of left atrium, corresponding to fossa ovalis of right atrium.

Q. What are the parts of the interventricular septum?

Ans. It's right side is convex and buldges into right ventricle. Greater part of septum is thick and muscular and small area near posterior margin is membranous.

Q. What is the developmental origin of ventricles?

Ans. The ventricles develop from:

(a) Bulbus cordis and

(b) Primitive ventricle.

Q. How interventricular septum develops?

Ans. (a) *Muscular part:* Upgrowth from apex of heart.

(b) *Membranous part:* Downgrowth from interatrial septum.

Q. What type of valves are present in heart?

Ans. (a) *Atrioventricular valves:* One pair

Right atrioventricular valve: Tricuspid valve, made up of three cusps.

Left atrioventricular valve: Bicuspid or mitral valve, made up of two cusps.

(b) *Semilunar valves:* One pair

Aortic and pulmonary valves. Each valve has 3 cusps.

Q. What is 'stenosis' of valve?

Ans. Narrowing of valve orifice due to fusion of valve cusps.

Q. What is 'incompetence' of valve?

Ans. The imperfect closure of the valve due to dilatation of valve orifice or stiffening of valve cusps.

Q. What are the septal defects?

Ans. These are the defects resulting from involvement of interatrial or interventricular septum.

1. Atrial septal defects include osteum secondum and osteum primum defects.
   An osteum secondum defect lies high up in the atrial wall, while the osteum primum defect lies below. These result in communication between left and right atria.

2. Interventricular septal defects which consist mainly of failure of development of membranous part. These are often associated with other septal defects.
3. Complete failure of a septum to form, resulting in formation of common atrium or common ventricle or both.

Q. What is dextrocardia?

Ans. This is a congenital anomaly in which the heart position is reversed and it lies on the right side of the thorax. This may be associated with the reversal of all the intra-abdominal organs (*situs inversus).*

Q. What will be the effect of pulmonary stenosis?

Ans. There will be right ventricular hypertrophy because heart tries to force blood through the narrowed valve. This will be associated with congestion in the right atrium followed by secondary right atrial hypertrophy.

Q. What is Fallot's tetralogy?

Ans. This is the commonest cyanotic congenital anomaly of the heart and consists of (1) pulmonary stenosis, (2) right ventricular hypertrophy, (3) venticular septal defect and (4) an overriding of the aorta over the septal defect. So, the aorta receives blood from both ventricles.

Q. What is complete transposition of great arteries?

Ans. It is a condition in which aorta arises from right ventricle and pulmonary trunk from left ventricle.

BLOOD SUPPLY OF HEART

Q. What is the origin of the right and left coronary arteries?

Ans.
1. The right coronary artery arises from the anterior aortic sinus. It is smaller than left.
2. The left coronary artery arises from the left posterior aortic sinus.

Q. What are the branches of the right coronary artery?

Ans.
1. Marginal branch,
2. Posterior (inferior) interventricular branch,
3. Nodal branch,

4. Right atrial branch,
5. Infundibular and
6. Terminal branches.

Q. What are the branches of the left coronary artery?

Ans. 1. Anterior interventricular branch.
2. Branch to diaphragmatic surface of left ventricle and
3. Left atrial branch.

The continuation of the left coronary artery after anterior interventricular branch is called the *circumflex artery*.

Q. What is the distribution of the right coronary artery?

Ans. 1. Large part of the right ventricle except area adjoining anterior interventricular groove.
2. Most of the right atrium.
3. Part of the left ventricle, near interventricular septum.
4. Posterior part of interventricular septum.
5. SA node in 60% of the cases.
6. AV node and Bundle of His except part of left branch of AV bundle.

Q. What is the distribution of the left coronary artery?

Ans. 1. Large part of the left ventricle
2. Right ventricle adjoining anterior interventricular groove
3. Left atrium
4. Anterior part of interventricular septum
5. SA node in 40% of the cases
6. Part of left branch of AV bundle.

Both the interatrial and interventricular septa are supplied by branches of both coronary arteries.

Q. Do the coronary arteries anastomose?

Ans. They anastomose to a slight extent. The interventricular branches of the two coronary arteries anastomose near the apex of the heart and in the interventricular septum. Coronary arteries also anastomose with vasa vasora of aorta, internal thoracic artery and bronchial arteries.

Q. What is the clinical importance of the anastomosis between the coronary arteries?

Ans. The anastomosis between the branches of the coronary arteries is inadequate to compensate for the sudden occlusion.

A blockage therefore leads to death (infarction) of the affected cardiac tissue.

Q. What is 'Angina pectoris'?

Ans. It is a clinical condition characterised by pain in front of the chest radiating to the ulnar side of the left arm and forearm. This is due to an incomplete obstruction of the coronary arteries.

Q. What are the tributaries of the coronary sinus?

Ans.
1. Great cardiac vein
2. Middle cardiac vein
3. Small cardiac vein
4. Oblique vein of the left atrium
5. Posterior vein of the left ventricle and
6. Right marginal vein.

Q. What are Thebsian veins?

Ans. These are small veins present in all chambers of heart opening directly into cavity of chambers.

Q. How is the coronary sinus developed?

Ans. The coronary sinus is developed from the left horn of the sinus venosus.

Q. Where does the coronary sinus open?

Ans. Into posterior wall of right atrium.

CONDUCTING SYSTEM OF THE HEART

Q. What are the functions of conducting system of heart?

Ans.
(a) It is responsible for initiating and maintaining normal cardiac rhythm.
(b) Ensures proper co-ordination of atrial and ventricular contractions.

Q. What is the sinuatrial (SA) node and where is it located?

Ans. The SA node is the pacemaker of the heart. It is situated in the right atrium along the anterior margin of opening of the superior vena cava.

Q. What is the position of AV node?

Ans. The AV node lies in the wall of right atrium formed by interatrial septum near the opening of the coronary sinus. It receives impulse from SA node.

Q. What is Atrioventricular bundle? What are its divisions?

Ans. AV bundle forms the connection between atrial and ventricular musculature. It begins at AV node and reaches posterior margin of membranous part of ventricular septum. Here it divides into left and right branches, which descend on left and right side of interventricular septum beneath endocardium. Each branch divides and subdivides to form Purkinje fibres, which terminate in ventricles.

Q. What are the histological differences between fibres of conducting system and cardiac muscle?

Ans. (a) Nodal fibres have more striations and are narrower than cardiac muscle fibres.

(b) Purkinje fibres are broader than myocardial fibres.

(c) These contain fewer organelles.

(d) Flasma membrane is thin.

(e) Desmosomes are more numerous.

Q. What is the 'moderator' band?

Ans. The 'moderator' band also called the *septomarginal trabecula* (one of the trabeculae carneae) extends from the ventricular septum to the anterior papillary muscle. This is important as it carries the right branch of the atrioventricular bundle (bundle of His). It may assist in preventing over distension of ventricle.

Q. What is the nerve supply of the heart?

Ans. Nerve supply to heart is by:

(a) Parasympathetic fibres via vagus nerve. These are cardioinhibitory.

(b) Sympathetic fibres from $T_{2\text{-}5}$ segments of spinal cord. There are cardioaccelerator and sensory. Both types of nerves form superficial and deep cardiac plexus and supply the heart.

Q. How is the superficial cardiac plexus formed? What are its branches?

Ans. The superficial cardiac plexus formed by:

(1) The inferior cervical cardiac branch of the left vagus and

(2) The superior cervical cardiac branch of left sympathetic trunk.

It is located just below the arch of aorta close to ligamentum arteriosum. It gives branches to deep cardiac plexus, right coronary artery and left pulmonary plexus.

Q. How is the deep cardiac plexus formed and what is its distribution?

Ans. The deep cardiac plexus is formed by:

(1) Cardiac branches of the both vagus.

(2) Cardiac branches of both recurrent laryngeal nerves and

(3) The cardiac branches of cervical and thoracic branches of sympathetic trunk

It gives branches to coronary and pulmonary plexuses and atria.

MAJOR BLOOD VESSELS OF THORAX

SUPERIOR VENA CAVA

Q. How superior vena cava is formed?

Ans. By the union of two brachiocephalic veins behind the lower border of first costal cartilage close to sternum.

Q. Name the tributaries of superior vena cava.

Ans. 1. Azygous vein,
2. Mediastinal veins and
3. Pericardial veins.

Q. What is the pathway for the collateral circulation in obstruction of superior vena cava?

Ans. (a) *If obstructed above opening of Azygous vein:* Venous blood from upper half of body is returned through azygous vein and superficial veins of chest are dilated upto costal margin.

(b) *If obstructed below opening of Azygous vein:* Venous blood is returned through inferior vena cava via femoral vein and superficial veins are dilated on chest and abdomen upto saphenous opening in thigh (Thoraco-epigastric vein).

Q. How superior vena cava is developed?

Ans. (a) *Upper half, upto opening of azygous vein:* Right anterior cardinal vein.

(b) *Lower half, below opening of azygous vein:* Right common cardinal vein.

PULMONARY TRUNK AND ARTERIES

Q. What is the course of pulmonary trunk?

Ans. It begins opposite the sternal end of left 3rd costal cartilage and upper end lies in front of fifth thoracic vertebra.

The bifurcation of pulmonary trunk lies below the arch of aorta.

Q. What are the relations of right pulmonary artery?

Ans. *Anterior:* Ascending aorta, Superior vena cava and Upper right pulmonary vein.

Posterior: Oesophagus and Right bronchus.

Q. What are the relations of left pulmonary artery?

Ans. *Posterior:* Left bronchus and Descending aorta.

Superiorly: Connected to arch of aorta by ligamentum arteriosum.

AORTA

Q. What are the parts of aorta in thorax?

Ans. (a) Ascending aorta,
(b) Arch of aorta and
(c) Descending thoracic aorta.

Q. What is the course of ascending aorta?

Ans. It begins at level of lower border of 3rd costal cartilage behind left half of sternum. It runs upwards, forwards and to right and continues as arch of aorta at sternal end of upper border of second right costal cartilage.

Q. What is Aortic sinus?

Ans. It is dilatation of vessel wall at root of aorta above each cusp of aortic valve.

Q. Name the branches of ascending aorta?

Ans. (a) *Right coronary artery:* From anterior aortic sinus.
(b) *Left coronary artery:* From left posterior aortic sinus.

Q. What is the level of beginning and termination of arch of aorta?

Ans. It begins behind upper border of 2nd right sternochondral joint (lower border of T_4) and ends at lower border of body of 4th thoracic vertebra on left side.
Thus it begins and ends at same level but it begins anteriorly and ends posteriorly.

Q. What are the posterior and to the right relations of arch of aorta?

Ans. From behind forwards these are:
(a) Vertebral columr
(b) Oesophagus
(c) Trachea
(d) Superior vena cava
(e) Thoracic duct
(f) Left recurrent laryngeal nerve
(g) Deep cardiac plexus.

Q. Name the branches of arch of aorta.

Ans. (a) *Brachiocephalic artery:* Divides into right common carotid and right subclavian artery.

(b) Left common carotid,
(c) Left subclavian.
(d) Thyroid ima } Occasionally
(e) Vertebral artery }

Q. Name branches of descending thoracic aorta.

Ans. (a) *Posterior intercostal arteries:* For 3rd-11th spaces, on both sides,
(b) *Subcostal arteries:* On both sides,
(c) Two left bronchial arteries,
(d) Oesophageal branches.
(e) Pericardial branches,
(f) Mediastinal branches and
(g) Superior phrenic.

Q. What is Aortic Aneurysm?

Ans. It is localised abnormal dilatation of aorta.

Q. What is Coarctation of Aorta?

Ans. It is the narrowing of aorta, occuring usually immediately beyond the origin of left subclavian artery.
It leads to hypertension above the narrowing e.g., arms, neck and head and hypotension below e.g., lower limb.

Q. What is the developmental origin of aorta?

Ans. (a) *Ascending aorta:* From truncus arteriosus.
(b) *Arch of aorta:*
1. From ventral part of aortic sac and its left horn and
2. Left fourth arch artery.

(c) *Descending aorta:*
1. From left dorsal aorta below attachment of fourth arch artery.
2. Fused median vessel.

Q. What is 'ductus arteriosus'?

Ans. It is communication present in fetal life connecting left pulmonary artery with aorta just distal to origin of left subclavian artery. After birth, it gets obliterated and forms ligamentum arteriosusm.

Q. What will happen if ductus arteriosus remains patent?

Ans. It causes progressive enlargement of left ventricle and pulmonary hypertension.

AZYGOUS AND HEMIZYGOUS VEINS

Q. How azygous vein is formed and terminates?

Ans. By the union of right ascending lumbar and right subcostal vein at level of T_{12} vertebra and terminates at level of T_4 vertebra into superior vena cava.

Q. Name the tributaries of azygous vein.

Ans.
1. Right posterior intercostal veins.
2. Right superior intercostal veins.
3. Hemiazygous veins: Present on left side and joins azygous vein at T_8 level.
4. Accessory hemiazygous vein: Present on left side and joins azygous vein at T_7 level.
5. Right bronchial veins.
6. Oesophageal veins.
7. Mediastinal and pericardial veins.
8. Right ascending lumbar veins.
9. Right subcostal vein.

Q. Name the tributaries of hemiazygous vein.

Ans. (a) 9th-11th left posterior intercostal veins.
(b) Left ascending lumbar vein.
(c) Left subcostal vein.

OESOPHAGUS

Q. What is the length of oesophagus?

Ans. 25 cm.

Q. What is the extent of oesophagus?

Ans. (a) It begins in neck at level of lower border of C_5 vertebra *i.e.* at lower border of cricoid cartilage.
(b) It ends in abdomen at level of lower border of T_{11} vertebra, at cardiac orifice of stomach.

Q. What are the 'Curvatures of oesophagus'?

Ans. Oesophagus shows.

(a) Two side to side curvatures towards left.
   1. At root of neck.
   2. Oesophageal opening in diaphragm.

(b) *Anteroposterior curvature:* Follows curvature of spine.

Q. What are the sites of oesophageal constrictions?

Ans. (a) *At its commencement:* 6 inches from incisor teeth.

(b) *Where it is crossed by aortic arch:* 9 inches from incisor teeth.

(c) *Where it is crossed by left bronchus:* 11 inches from incisor teeth.

(d) *At its termination:* 15 inches from incisor teeth.

Q. Name the structures intervening between oesophagus and vertebral column.

Ans. 1. Thoracic duct
2. Vena azygos
3. Hemiazygos vein
4. Accessory hemiazygos vein
5. Right posterior intercostal arteries.

Q. What are the divisions of oesophagus?

Ans. The oesophagus is divided into three parts:

(a) Cervical,
(b) Thoracic and
(c) Abdominal.

Q. What is the relation of recurrent laryngeal newes to the oesophagus in the neck?

Ans. The right and left recurrent laryngeal newes lie anterolateral to the oesophagus in corresponding grooves between it and the trachea.

Q. What is the blood supply of oesophagus?

Ans. *Arterial supply:*

(a) *Cervical part:* Inferior thyroid artery.

(b) *Thoracic part:* Oesophageal branches of aorta and bronchial arteries.

(c) *Abdominal part:* Oesophageal branches of left gastric artery.

Venous drainage:

(a) *Cervical part:* Into brachiocephalic vein.

(b) *Thoracic part:* Into azygous vein.

(c) *Abdominal part:* Into portal vein through left gastric vein. Lower end is site of porto-systemic anastomosis.

Q. What is the nerve supply of oesophagus?

Ans. *Parasympathetic nerves:*

Sensorimotor and secretomotor.

Upper ½: Recurrent laryngeal nerve.

Lower ½: Oesophageal plexus formed by two vagus nerves.

Sympathetic nerves:

Vasomotor.

Upper ½: Fibres from middle cervical ganglion.

Lower ½: Fibres from upper 4 thoracic ganglia.

Q. What is 'Achalasia cardia'?

Ans. It is condition of neuromuscular incoordination in which the lower end of oesophagus fails to dilate when food is swallowed. As a result, food accumulates in the oesophagus.

Q. What is the clinical importance of constrictions of oesophagus?

Ans. 1. During endoscopy, these constrictions should be kept in mind.

2. These are also the sites of development of strictures usually.

Q. What are oesophageal varices and what is their clinical importance?

Ans. These are the dilatations of the oesophageal veins in portal hypertension, which form anastomosis between azygos (systemic) and left gastric (portal) veins.

Clinical importance: These may rupture leading to severe haemorrhage.

Q. What is the effect of enlargement of left atrium on oesophagus?

Ans. In mitral stenosis, enlargement of left atrium causes backward displacement of the oesophagus, which can be seen in a barium swallow.

Q. How oesophagus is developed?

Ans. The oesophagus is developed from the part of foregut lying between pharynx and stomach. It is at first short but later on elongates with the descent of diaphragm and formation of neck.

Q. What are the characteristic histological features of oesophagus?

Ans. From within outwards it is made up of:

(a) *Mucosa:* Lined by stratified squamous epithelium.
(b) *Submucosa:* Contains mucous glands.
(c) *Muscular layer:* Has external longitudinal and inner circular fibres. The muscle fibres are striated in upper two thirds and smooth in lower one third.
(d) Connective tissue sheath of areolar tissue.

Q. What are the common congenital abnormalities of oesophagus?

Ans. (a) Atresia with or without tracheo-oesophageal fistula.
(b) *Stenosis:* Narrowing of lumen of oesophagus.
(c) Short oesophagus.

THORACIC DUCT

Q. What is the length of thoracic duct?

Ans. 40 cm.

Q. What is the extent of thoracic duct?

Ans. Begins from Cisterna chyli near lower border of T_{12} vertebra. Ends into angle of junction between left subclavian and left internal jugular vein at level of T_2 vertebra.

Q. What are the relations of thoracic duct in aortic opening of diaphragm?

Ans. (a) *Anteriorly:* Diaphragm
(b) *Posteriorly:* Vertebral column
(c) *To the left:* Azygous vein
(d) *To the right:* Aorta.

Q. Name the tributaries of thoracic duct.

Ans. *In thorax:*

(a) Channels from posterior mediastinal and intercostal nodes.

(b) Left mediastinal trunk may drain.

At root of neck:

(a) Left jugular trunk,

(b) Left subclavian trunk.

Q. From which areas the thoracic duct drains lymph?

Ans. (a) Both halves of body below diaphragm and

(b) Left half above diaphragm.

SYMPATHETIC TRUNK

Q. What is the extent of sympathetic trunk?

Ans. Each trunk is placed on either side of vertebral column and extends from base of skull to coccyx below.

Q. What is the position of sympathetic trunk in relation to vertebral column?

Ans. *In cervical region:* Anterior to transverse processes of cervical vertebrae.

In thoracic region: Anterior to heads of ribs

In lumbar region: Anterolateal to lumbar vertebrae.

In sacral region: Anterior to sacrum.

The two join each other in front of the coccyx.

Q. What is the number of ganglia in cervical sympathetic trunk?

Ans. Three

Q. What is ganglion impar?

Ans. The lower fused ends of right and left sympathetic trunks are thickened in a midline ganglion called as ganglion impar.

Q. Where the cell body of sympathetic preganglionic neurons are present?

Ans. In the intermedio-lateral grey column of spinal cord in spinal segment T_1 to L_2.

Q. What is the location of sympathetic post ganglionic neurons?

Ans. Ganglia on sympathetic trunk.

Q. What is the number of ganglia in thoracic sympathetic trunk?

Ans. 12, but may be reduced due to fusion of adjacent ganglia with one another.

Q. What is 'stellate ganglion'?

Ans. It is ganglion formed by fusion of first thoracic ganglion with inferior cervical ganglion.

Q. Name the branches of thoracic part of sympathetic trunk.

Ans. *Lateral branches:*

Each ganglion is connected with corresponding spinal nerve, by white (preganglionic) and grey (postganglionic) rami communicans.

Medial branches:

(a) Pulmonary branches to pulmonary plexus (b) Cardiac branches to cardiac plexus (c) Aortic branches to arotic plexus (d) Oesophageal branches to oesophageal plexus	From upper five ganglia.
(e) *Greater splanchnic nerve:* By roots from ganglia 5 to 9. Ends mainly in coeliac ganglion (f) *Lesser splanchnic nerve:* By roots from ganglia 10 and 11. Ends mainly in aorticorenal ganglia. (g) *Least splanchnic nerve:* By roots of ganglion 12. Ends in renal plexus.	Preganglionic from lower seven ganglia.

PHRENIC NERVES

Q. How the phrenic nerve is formed?

Ans. Each nerve is formed by ventral primary rami of C_3, C_4 and C_5 spinal nerves. The contribution from C_4 is greatest.

Q. What is the distribution of the phrenic nerve?

Ans. *Motor:* To diaphragm.

Sensory:

1. Proprioceptive fibres from diaphragm
2. Sensory branches to pericardium and parietal pleura.
3. Sensory branches to suprarenal glands, inferior vena cava and gall bladder.